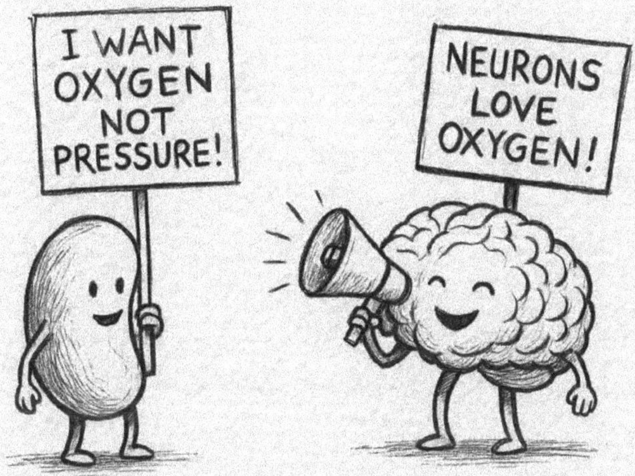

Currency of Care: Oxygen Delivery in the PCICU

Rohit S. Loomba, MD
loombabooks@gmail.com

Thanks to Yaeji Kim of CHD doodles for her wonderful

For free, specimen-based cardiac anatomy videos of congenitally malformed hearts visit the link below!

For a specimen-based cardiac anatomy textbook with images of actual hearts visit the link below!

Table of contents

1. Introduction 4
2.The oximetric framework 7
3. Oximetric indices and monitoring 25
4. Medical and procedural interventions 45
5. Cardiopulmonary bypass and its effects 53
6. Circulatory physiologies 59
7. Fully septated biventricular physiology 61
8. Left to right shunt physiology 63
9. Limitation to pulmonary blood flow physiology 70
10. Limitation to systemic blood flow physiology 77
11. Transposition physiology 85
12. Functionally univentricular physiologies 93
13. Ventricular dysfunction physiologies 105
14. Respiratory support and cardiopulmonary interactions 109
15. Venous circulation 113
16. The oximetric framework in practice 120

1
Introduction

The pediatric cardiac intensive care unit is a complex environment. Critically ill children, and even adults, are often cared for in both the medical and surgical contexts. This is all done in the setting of a unit in which there are a variety of faculty and staff who must work together with one another as well as with the patients and their families.

What makes the pediatric cardiac intensive care unit truly unique is that congenital heart disease often results in abnormal circulatory patterns, all of which may respond differently to specific interventions and differently according to age. The multiple levels of variability lead to highly complex medical situations, especially in the presence of insufficiency or failure in multiple organ systems.

The complexity of what is being managed in the pediatric cardiac intensive care unit requires a measured and tempered approach. The approach must be holistic and include monitoring strategies, review of monitoring data, interpretation of monitoring data, understanding of available interventions, and selection of interventions. Any approach cannot be linear and must be circular such that the process is repeated periodically to effectively risk stratify patients for morbidity and mortality and allow for early intervention.

The goal of this text is to provide a concise overview of core principles fundamental to providing care in the cardiac intensive care unit. This will be done using an oximetric based approach in which monitoring of, and maintenance of, regional and systemic oxygen delivery will be the focus. This approach's benefits over other approaches, such as pressure-based approaches will be discussed. Additionally, the limitations of such an approach will be discussed as well.

This is meant to be a concise text focused on global principles which can then be supplemented with more detailed texts. This does mean certain topics may not be covered at all or may just be covered briefly. Additionally, to keep the text relatively compact and easy to read it was elected not to include references within each chapter. All readers are encouraged to "trust but verify". Readers are encouraged to seek references to support discussed concepts. Some references are provided at the end of this text. Readers may feel free to contact the author to request additional supporting data.

This text will not cover psychosocial dynamics in the pediatric cardiac intensive care unit. This is not to imply these are not important but rather to imply that psychosocial dynamics are complex and require more specific focus than can be provided by this text.

Hopefully this text is helpful in providing a framework with which to approach clinical management in the pediatric cardiac intensive care unit. Each patient is unique and there will never be a single management algorithm. What there can be, however, is a single thought algorithm. That is the purpose of this text; to provide a useful framework with which to approach clinical monitoring and management in the cardiac intensive care unit using an oximetric method. These principles apply across units despite the focus of this textbook being the pediatric cardiac intensive care unit.

While the approach outlined in this text is intuitive and evidence-based, it does represent a departure from conventional textbooks.

2
The oximetric framework

The oximetric approach

A systematic, reproducible approach is necessary when approaching any situation. The care of a pediatric cardiac intensive care patient is no different, although one could argue that the need for a systematic, reproducible approach is greater in this setting. In this setting, an approach to clinical care must include a starting framework of thought, identification of clinical indices to monitor, a strategy for monitoring these clinical indices, and a system by which to decide whether the clinical indices indicate the need for a change in clinical interventions. Often in clinical practice, the aims or clinical indices to target appear to change without respect to a single overarching aim.

To establish a framework, it is necessary to establish the goals of clinical care in the pediatric cardiac intensive care unit. It is reasonable to propose that the primary aim is to help facilitate clinical improvement while minimizing morbidity and mortality. It then becomes necessary to define "clinical improvement". It is here that things can often become contested amongst clinicians or even change with time for the same clinician.

But perhaps nature can help inform us in this regard. The basic need of the body and its constituent organs is the need for oxygen. Without oxygen the body cannot create adenosine triphosphate and bodily functions will cease. Bearing testament to this is the fact that the human body has evolved several systems that focus on the uptake of oxygen and its delivery across the body. The airways are responsible for drawing in oxygen-containing air with help from the respiratory muscles including the diaphragm. The lungs then help diffuse oxygen from the inhaled air into the circulating blood, which serves as a carrier for oxygen. Oxygen-containing blood is then pumped to the constituent organs for them to extract oxygen for use by individual cells to produce adenosine triphosphate and fuel cellular processes that maintain larger body-wide processes. The heart serves as a pump to help provide a kinetic force that aids in the propulsion of oxygen-containing blood. Once the organs extract oxygen, de-oxygenated blood must return to the lungs to be re-oxygenated. And so, the cycle continues.

This is not to say other vital processes, such as the elimination of carbon dioxide and other cellular byproducts, aren't also important, but it is to highlight that without oxygen none of these other processes can be maintained for meaningful amounts of time. Certainly, anaerobic mechanisms for energy production exist in the body but these merely serve as temporary measures until the primary aerobic mechanisms can be re-established. If the aerobic mechanisms of energy production cannot be re-established, then the anaerobic mechanisms will rapidly become inadequate in producing enough energy to sustain cellular processes.

Adequacy of oxygen delivery

The maintenance of adequate oxygen delivery is thus of utmost importance. The adequacy of oxygen delivery is mediated by oxygen delivery and oxygen extraction. Oxygen delivery is influenced by the amount of oxygen that is inhaled, the amount of oxygen that is dissolved and bound in the blood, the amount of oxygen-containing blood that is pumped by the heart, the regional distribution of pumped oxygen-containing blood, the ability of the organs to extract oxygen, and the amount of oxygen the organs are utilizing.

Adequacy of oxygen delivery is a regional phenomenon, and a variety of factors influence regional oxygen delivery. It is important to note that the notion of "global'' oxygen delivery can be falsely reassuring. For instance, global oxygen delivery may seem adequate with a preserved systemic venous saturation but there may be regional cerebral inadequacy of oxygen delivery in the setting of a thrombotic cerebral stroke. There is a growing body of evidence regarding the implications of regional oxygen delivery. Adequacy, or rather inadequacy, of oxygen delivery has been demonstrated to be associated with cerebral stroke, neurodevelopment delay, vision loss in retinal occlusion, need for intubation, cardiac dysfunction, hepatic insufficiency, acute kidney injury, necrotizing enterocolitis, and limb ischemia among other morbidities. Thus, regional venous saturations can be helpful.

Oxygen delivery

If oxygen is the key to cellular function, it then becomes relatively intuitive that oxygen delivery is what should be monitored and maintained. This requires an understanding of what oxygen delivery is, objectively. Oxygen delivery is the product of oxygen content and cardiac output.

Oxygen content, specifically, is the sum of the bound and dissolved components of oxygen. The bound component represents the amount of oxygen bound to hemoglobin and generally is most of the oxygen content. Dissolved oxygen represents a small fraction of oxygen content but should not be ignored, particularly at high fractions of inspired oxygen. The first half of the equation, as written below, quantifies the bound component of oxygen and consists of the maximum amount of oxygen that can be bound to hemoglobin, the oxygen saturation which is the percent of hemoglobin sites bound by oxygen, and then the amount of hemoglobin. The second half of the equation, as written below, quantifies the dissolved component of oxygen and consists of a constant and then the partial pressure of oxygen.

$$Oxygen\ content = (1.36\ x\ oxygen\ saturation\ x\ hemoglobin) + (0.003\ x\ partial\ pressure\ of\ oxygen)$$

The equation is purposely written without specifying a circulatory bed such as arterial, capillary, or venous. This is because oxygen content can be calculated for any circulatory bed by using the values specific to that circulatory bed. From the equation it becomes clear that oxygen content can be augmented by increasing oxygen saturation, hemoglobin, or the partial pressure of oxygen.

Cardiac output is best quantified by the Fick principle. This principle essentially uses oxygen as an indicator and calculates a volume of cardiac output by dividing oxygen consumption by the arteriovenous oxygen content difference.

$$Cardiac\ ouput = \frac{Oxygen\ consumption}{Arterial\ oxygen\ content - venous\ oxygen\ content}$$

The equation makes it clear that cardiac output tends to increase with an increase in oxygen consumption and that cardiac output increases with a decrease in the arteriovenous oxygen content difference.

The product of oxygen content and cardiac output then allows for quantification of oxygen delivery. But apart from quantifying the amount of oxygen delivery, these equations help provide a logical framework to approach the optimization of oxygen delivery. Oxygen content is relatively intuitive to follow as its components are discrete. Cardiac output is less intuitive to follow as oxygen consumption is not easily monitored, although it can be estimated. To better conceptualize cardiac output, it is better to treat cardiac output as the product of heart rate and stroke volume. Stroke volume can further be broken down into its mediators of preload, afterload, and contractility.

As a result of this, oxygen delivery is found to be mediated by oxygen content, heart rate, preload, afterload, and contractility.

Oxygen extraction

As the adequacy of oxygen delivery is based on both oxygen delivery and oxygen extraction, decreasing oxygen extraction can be helpful in optimizing the adequacy of oxygen delivery.

Myocardial oxygen extraction may be increased for several reasons, with tachycardia being one such reason. Controlling the rate or controlling fever that may be leading to tachycardia may help decrease myocardial oxygen extraction. Particularly at high rates there may be a significant increase in myocardial oxygen consumption.

Global oxygen extraction also increases in the setting of infection, independent of fever as a mechanism.

Thus, controlling infection, whether bacterial or viral is of great importance.

Enteral feeds can also lead to increased oxygen extraction with both continuous and bolus enteral feeds potentially increasing oxygen extraction. Close monitoring of the adequacy of systemic oxygen delivery is important when enteral feeds are being initiated or advanced in critically ill children. Holding feeds or slowly advancing feeds can help minimize oxygen extraction.

Pain, agitation, and discomfort can also lead to increased oxygen extraction. This is mediated by resulting tachycardia but also the associated voluntary muscle activity in response to the unwanted stimuli. Apart from patient comfort, pain control is also important in minimizing oxygen extraction.

Respiratory distress can also lead to a significant increase in oxygen extraction. The respiratory muscles can extract over a third of circulating oxygen in the setting of severe respiratory distress, and escalation of respiratory support can be helpful in reducing oxygen extraction.

Analgesia, sedation, paralysis, infection control, modulation of feeds, and intubation are all thus helpful tools in minimizing oxygen extraction and contribute to improving the adequacy of oxygen delivery.

Oxygen content

In addition to minimizing oxygen extraction, it is important to maximize oxygen delivery. The components of oxygen delivery have already been discussed. Oxygen content may be augmented by increasing hemoglobin levels or increasing the fraction of inspired oxygen.

Transfusion of packed red blood cells has been demonstrated to increase oxygen delivery. Studies have demonstrated, particularly in postoperative cardiac patients with inadequate oxygen delivery, that transfusion of packed red blood cells can improve oxygen delivery. Such transfusions may have variable impact depending on the circulatory physiology. Physiology-specific considerations will be discussed later.

Oxygen content

Increasing the fraction of inspired oxygen can help improve oxygen delivery by increasing the oxygen saturation and the partial pressure of oxygen. The arterial saturation can be monitored by pulse oximetry or blood gas analysis while the partial pressure of oxygen can be monitored by blood gas analysis.

Cardiac output components- heart rate, preload, afterload, contractility

Cardiac output can be optimized by increasing heart rate, increasing preload, decreasing afterload, and/or increasing contractility.

Heart rate is relatively intuitive. Increasing heart rate is generally associated with an increase in cardiac output if atrioventricular synchrony is maintained. At higher heart rates there is a decrease in diastolic filling time, and this can eventually lead to impairment in stroke volume. Thus, after some heart rate there will no longer be an increase in stroke volume with increasing heart rate. Eventually, there may even be a decrease in stroke volume. Stroke volume, however, is preserved across a large range of heart rates.

Heart rate can be augmented by electrical pacing or by chronotropic agents. Electrical pacing can be achieved by transesophageal pacing or by wires placed on the heart. Chemical pacing may be achieved by chronotropic agents including, but not limited, to isoproterenol, epinephrine, norepinephrine, dopamine, or dobutamine. There are no real defined thresholds for heart rate at which cardiac output is optimized, and such a threshold is variable across patients.

Along with heart rate, heart rhythm is also important. Loss of atrioventricular synchrony can greatly impact cardiac output. Cardiac output can decrease approximately 30% with loss of atrioventricular synchrony, particularly in functionally univentricular physiologies.

Preload is the amount of force exerted upon the myocyte at end diastole. Often preload is equated to the volume of blood in the ventricle at end diastole but that is not accurate. Preload is a loading phenomenon which is a force and not a volume. This net force on the ventricular myocytes is multivectoral, being exerted on the myocytes from inside the ventricular cavity and from outside the heart. Such a force is best described by the law of Laplace.

$$Ventricular\ preload = \frac{end\ diastolic\ pressure\ x\ end\ diastolic\ radius}{2\ x\ wall\ thickness}$$

The equation can be used for either ventricle and this equation makes it objectively clear that ventricular preload is not equal to end diastolic volume. Loads are forces and not volumes. Treating the two synonymously is not only scientifically inaccurate but also offers no clinical benefit. If one wishes to refer to end diastolic volume, then there's no need to call it by any other name.

The equation's numerator is the product of end diastolic pressure and end diastolic radius and serves as a marker of compliance. In the setting of greater ventricular compliance, end diastolic radius will be greater at a given end diastolic pressure. Thus, ventricular compliance influences preload and greater compliance is associated with greater stroke volume and cardiac output. The denominator of the equation is twice the ventricular wall thickness; thus, the greater the wall thickness the lower the stroke volume or cardiac output.

A more compliant ventricle with greater end diastolic pressure and greater end diastolic radius allows for optimal preload as increasing preload facilitates greater myocyte contraction. This increase is not linear. If preload is plotted on the x-axis and stroke volume on the y-axis, stroke volume increases in a convex fashion with increasing preload until a point where stroke volume plateaus. It should be noted that this relationship is often attributed to Frank and Starling. Their independent experiments utilized end diastolic volume as a surrogate for preload, and as discussed before, end diastolic volume and preload are not interchangeable. Repeat experiments using end diastolic pressure have also shown similar findings.

This construct of preload is evident in the setting or hypertrophic cardiomyopathy. Decreased ventricular compliance results in higher end diastolic pressure and lower end diastolic radius, resulting in a lower value for the numerator in the preload equation.

Decreased ventricular compliance also leads to increased wall thickness, resulting in a high value of the denominator in the preload equation. A low numerator and high denominator results in a low value for preload, a state associated with lower stroke volume.

Ventricular preload is difficult to monitor clinically. The equation explicitly indicates what would need to be monitored. It simply is not practical to measure these values serially in an intensive care unit, particularly not continuously.

Augmenting preload, clinically, can be accomplished by improving ventricular compliance and/or providing a fluid bolus. Medications that may improve ventricular compliance in children include angiotensin converting enzyme inhibitors, angiotensin receptor blockers, beta blockers, and calcium channel blockers. These all can take time to have a true effect on ventricular compliance. Levosimendan and milrinone may have indirect effects on ventricular compliance that may be beneficial, but these also take time. Augmenting preload by providing a fluid bolus is also an option. This will help increase the end diastolic pressure and end diastolic radius product and, thus, preload.

Similar to preload, afterload is a force. It is the amount of force exerted on the myocyte at end systole. Often afterload is equated to arterial blood pressure, but loads are forces and not pressures. An interesting logical predicament also arises with the oversimplification of preload and afterload as preload is often equated to a volume while afterload is often equated to a pressure. Afterload, similar to preload, is multivectoral. It represents the force that the heart must overcome for blood to be ejected. Afterload is also best described using the law of Laplace.

$$Ventricular\ afterload = \frac{end\ systolic\ pressure\ x\ end\ systolic\ radius}{2\ x\ wall\ thickness}$$

This equation can be used for either ventricle and makes it objectively clear that ventricular afterload is not equal to arterial blood pressure. Loads are forces and not pressures. Treating the two synonymously is not only scientifically inaccurate but also offers no clinical benefit. If one wishes to refer to arterial blood pressure, then there's no need to call it by any other name.

The numerator in the afterload equation is the product of end systolic pressure and end systolic radius. A lower end systolic pressure and end systolic radius product implies less wall stress and less force opposing the myocytes. The denominator in the equation is, once again, twice the wall thickness. Greater systolic wall thickness is associated with lower afterload which is then associated with greater stroke volume.

Thus, at end systole, low systolic pressure, low end systolic radius, and greater wall thickness are associated with lower afterload and greater stroke volume.

Similar to ventricular preload, afterload is also not practical to monitor in an intensive care unit. The equation makes it clear what would need to be measured but these values are not easily measured, particularly not simultaneously or continuously.

Afterload can be reduced in the clinical setting by using medications such as angiotensin converting enzyme inhibitors, angiotensin receptor blockers, calcium channel blockers, sodium nitroprusside, nicardipine, hydralazine, beta blockers, milrinone, or levosimendan. Positive pressure ventilation can also help reduce left ventricular afterload.

It is important to note that interventions may have different direction and magnitude of effect on preload and afterload for the right and left ventricle.

The final mediator of cardiac output is contractility. This the amount a myocyte contracts. As contractility increases, cardiac output increases. The contractile elements, the process of contraction itself, and the factors influencing this contraction are beyond the scope of this text. Inotropes such as epinephrine, norepinephrine, dopamine, dobutamine, isoproterenol, milrinone, and levosimendan can help improve myocyte contractility.

Component	Subcomponents	Clinical interventions
Oxygen Content	Hb, SaO_2, PaO_2	Transfusion, FiO_2
Cardiac Output	HR, Preload, Afterload, Contractility	Pacing, fluids, inotropes, vasodilators

Blood pressure

Clinical care is often titrated to arterial blood pressure. Arterial blood pressure can be clinically monitored noninvasively using a blood pressure cuff and invasively using an arterial line. The former provides intermittent monitoring while the latter provides continuous monitoring.

But what is arterial blood pressure and what does it actually convey? The pressure in any liquid containing system is equal to the product of flow and resistance. In the setting of arterial blood pressure this is equal to the product of systemic blood flow and systemic vascular resistance. In the clinical setting, arterial blood pressure is often equated to systemic blood flow and increases in arterial blood pressure are assumed to represent increases in systemic blood flow, while decreases in arterial blood pressure are assumed to represent decreases in systemic blood flow. However, this assumption is flawed. An increase in arterial blood pressure may simply be secondary to an increase in systemic vascular resistance. Similarly, a decrease in blood pressure may be due to a decrease in systemic vascular resistance. An increase in arterial blood pressure may occur with a decrease in systemic blood flow but a concomitant increase in systemic vascular resistance of greater magnitude. A decrease in arterial blood pressure may occur with an increase in systemic blood flow but a concomitant decrease in systemic vascular resistance of greater magnitude.

Thus, assumptions regarding systemic blood flow based on arterial blood pressure are fraught with error if concurrent changes in systemic vascular resistance are not known. And unfortunately, systemic vascular resistance is not easily monitored in routine clinical practice. Pressure-based titration of care may lead to use of agents that increase systemic vascular resistance without increasing systemic blood flow or even decreasing it. This is problematic as systemic blood flow and not systemic vascular resistance is what is oxygen-containing, and it is oxygen that the organs need. In fact, increasing systemic vascular resistance may lead to decrease in stroke volume and oxygen delivery. This has been demonstrated in functionally univentricular and biventricular circulatory physiologies in pediatric patients.

Arterial blood pressure has been monitored in various fashions since the late 1700s, but the first blood gas analyzer was not developed until 1957. Because of the longer experience with blood pressure, it has become engrained in clinical practice. However, history should not be allowed to overpower science and objective data. If oxygen and not pressure is what the body and its constituent organs need, then it is more logical that oximetric indices are used to titrate care rather than pressure indices. Historic practices and group think can be detrimental and have led to medical practices such as bloodletting to have sustained for over 3,000 years.

Additionally, upon review of the equations that describe oxygen delivery it becomes apparent that none of these equations include arterial blood pressure.

There are data that demonstrate the greater prognostic value of oximetric indices compared to blood pressure in most clinical settings. The benefits extend to the risk stratification of various morbidities and mortality across circulatory physiologies.

Vascular resistance

Vascular resistance is an important physiologic concept to understand. Vascular resistance is the force that opposes blood flow in a circulation. In humans, there are two primary resistances that are discussed- systemic and pulmonary vascular resistances.

$$Systemic\ vascular\ resistance = \frac{mean\ arterial\ pressure\ -\ central\ venous\ pressure}{systemic\ blood\ flow}$$

$$Pulmonary\ vascular\ resistance = \frac{pulmonary\ arterial\ pressure\ -\ pulmonary\ venous\ pressure}{pulmonary\ blood\ flow}$$

The equation for systemic vascular resistance highlights that systemic vascular resistance is not equal to mean arterial blood pressure nor is it equal to left ventricular afterload. Pulmonary vascular resistance is not equal to mean pulmonary artery pressure nor is it equal to right ventricular afterload. These are all distinctly different physiologic concepts and should be treated as such.

Clinical application of the oximetric framework

The oximetric framework hinges on the monitoring of oximetric indices. These will be discussed in detail later. But either the arteriovenous oxygen saturation difference or oxygen extraction can be utilized. In patients with baseline hypoxemia, such as those with functionally univentricular multidistributive physiology or Glenn physiology, oxygen extraction outperforms the arteriovenous oxygen saturation difference in risk stratification of morbidity and mortality.

$$Arteriovenous\ oxygen\ saturation\ difference = arterial\ oxygen\ saturation - venous\ oxygen\ saturation$$

$$Oxygen\ extraction = \frac{(arterial\ oxygen\ saturation - venous\ oxygen\ saturation)}{arterial\ oxygen\ saturation}$$

An arteriovenous oxygen saturation difference of 30 to 40 and an oxygen extraction of 30% to 40% is where the risk of morbidity and mortality increases. It is reasonable to use either as an assessment of the adequacy of oxygen delivery. If oxygen delivery is deemed inadequate by either metric, then escalations of care can be guided by utilizing the oximetric framework and assessing whether the inadequacy of oxygen delivery is believed to be due to increased oxygen extraction and/or decreased oxygen delivery. Then the individual components of each such as fraction of inspired oxygen, hemoglobin, heart rate, preload, afterload, and contractility can be assessed.

Once interventions are made then the same metric can be used to assess the efficacy of the intervention. And, conversely, if the arteriovenous oxygen saturation difference or oxygen extraction is reassuring then further interventions may not be required and support may even be weaned.

Limitations of the oximetric framework

As will be discussed later, oximetric monitoring requires monitoring the arterial and venous oxygen saturations, directly by blood gas analysis or indirectly with spectroscopy. In settings where the organs cannot extract oxygen, such as in organ death or some phenotypes of distributive shock, the venous saturation may be spuriously high. While the initial assumption would be that there is adequate oxygen delivery, the organs in these situations are simply not extracting oxygen.

In the setting of distributive shock phenotypes where the organs are unable to extract oxygen, the risk of morbidity and mortality is exceptionally high. Studies have demonstrated that lactate clearance, not absolute lactate nor blood pressure, have the most prognostic value in these settings.

The number of patients in the pediatric cardiac intensive care unit in whom the oximetric approach will not provide appropriate clinical guidance is low. It's also important to note that blood pressure does not offer additional prognostic value in these settings.

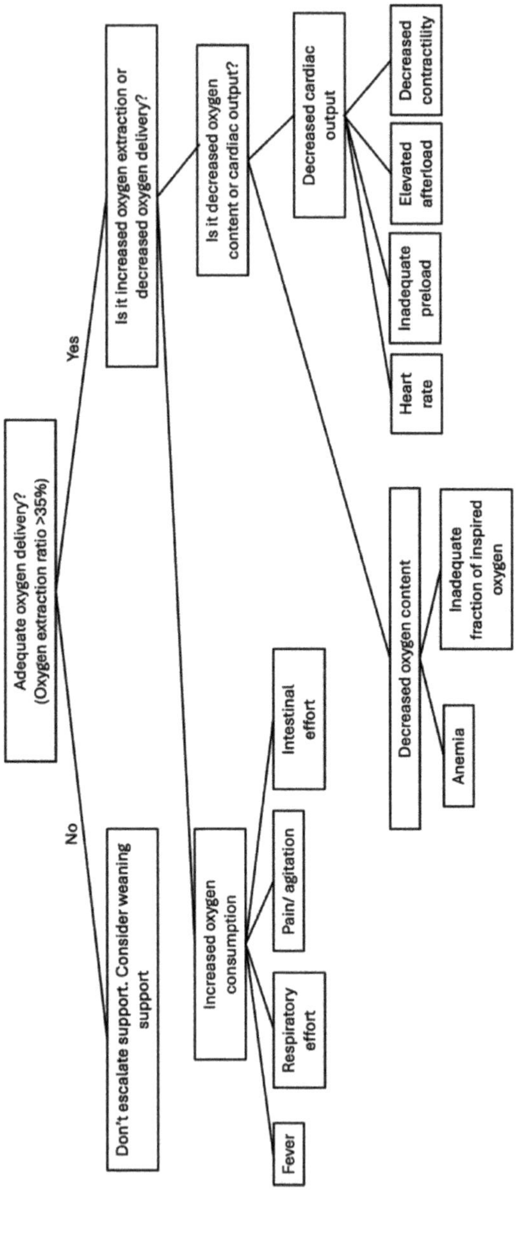
Adequate oxygen delivery?
(Oxygen extraction ratio >35%)
Yes
No
Is it increased oxygen extraction or decreased oxygen delivery?
Don't escalate support. Consider weaning support
Is it decreased oxygen content or cardiac output?
Increased oxygen consumption
Decreased cardiac output
Decreased oxygen content
Decreased contractility
Elevated afterload
Inadequate preload
Heart rate
Inadequate fraction of inspired oxygen
Anemia
Intestinal effort
Pain/ agitation
Respiratory effort
Fever

3
Oximetric indices and monitoring

Any approach to the assessment of critically ill patients and titration of clinical care must be based on adequate monitoring. Considerations specific to monitoring while using the oximetric framework are reviewed in this chapter. This is not meant to be an entirely exhaustive review of monitoring in a pediatric cardiac intensive care unit but rather a concise overview of monitoring pertinent to titrating clinical care using the oximetric framework. Monitoring should be patient, and setting, specific and aim to maximize efficiency of resource utilization and minimize patient discomfort.

Oximetric indices

The most important consideration when employing the oximetric framework is to monitor the venous oxygen saturation. The Fick principle makes it evident that cardiac output decreases as the difference between the arterial oxygen saturation and venous oxygen saturation increases. Conversely, cardiac output increases as the difference between the arterial oxygen saturation and venous oxygen saturation decreases. Thus, monitoring and trending the arteriovenous oxygen saturation difference is of importance. In addition to the arteriovenous oxygen saturation difference there is also oxygen extraction which is the arteriovenous oxygen saturation difference divided by the arterial saturation. In patients who are not fully saturated this can lead to a significant difference in assessment, while in those who are fully saturated on the arterial side the two metrics will be equal. In those with functionally univentricular multidistributive physiology, oxygen extraction has been shown to have greater prognostic ability although both perform well.

Arterial saturation – blood gas analysis and pulse oximetry

Monitoring the arterial oxygen saturation is routine practice. Arterial oxygen saturation is a component of the oxygen content, cardiac output, and oxygen delivery equations. Arterial oxygen saturation can directly be measured by arterial blood gas analysis or be estimated using pulse oximetry. Arterial blood gas analysis allows for precise quantification of the arterial oxygen saturation and also provides additional information but requires an arterial blood draw or an arterial line. Pulse oximetry is relatively inexpensive, widely available, and noninvasive. The estimate provided by pulse oximetry can be less accurate depending on skin tone and with lower arterial oxygen saturation.

There is no discrete cutoff for arterial oxygen saturation. The hemoglobin oxygen dissociation curve does have an inflection point which usually occurs at an arterial oxygen saturation between 88% and 92%. Thus, for those with biventricular circulation this is often used as a target for arterial oxygen saturation. It should be noted that a patient-specific cutoff for arterial oxygen saturation can be established by noting when oxygen delivery becomes inadequate. Obviously if it already is inadequate then augmenting the arterial oxygen saturation may prove to be helpful.

Venous saturation – blood gas analysis and near infrared spectroscopy

Monitoring venous oxygen saturation is less frequently done compared to arterial oxygen saturation. Venous oxygen saturation is a component of the oxygen content, cardiac output, and oxygen delivery equations. Venous oxygen saturation can be directly measured by venous blood gas analysis or be estimated using near infrared spectroscopy. Venous blood gas analysis allows for precise quantification of the venous oxygen saturation and can also provide additional information but requires a venous blood draw or a venous line. Near infrared spectroscopy offers a noninvasive means by which to estimate the underlying venous oxygen saturation. It is noninvasive and cheap over longer durations of time as the disposable sensors are not particularly expensive although they cost more than pulse oximetry sensors. The upfront cost for the monitors and initial supply of sensors can be expensive. The cost of the monitor, however, is diluted over time.

Near infrared spectroscopy utilizes separate wavelengths of light and light absorption to estimate the venous oxygen saturation. There are several monitors and sensors available through a few different manufacturers. They utilize different sized sensors with variable adhesive properties. They also employ different algorithms and may have variable sensitivity to changes in the underlying venous saturation. Bilirubin levels and skin tone can impact near infrared spectroscopy values. Some makes and models of near infrared spectroscopy monitors and sensors adjust for these factors more efficiently.

Whether the venous oxygen saturation is measured or estimated, the question is where to monitor the venous oxygen saturation. Historically, the mixed venous saturation has been considered most clinically valuable. However, this is not based on any substantial data. Additionally, in children with congenitally malformed hearts there may not be a true mixed venous saturation. This is particularly evident in functionally univentricular multidistributive physiology.

Studies have investigated simultaneously drawn samples from the superior and inferior caval vein in those with functionally univentricular and biventricular physiologies, demonstrating that both the superior caval vein oxygen saturation and the inferior caval vein oxygen saturation were significantly associated with morbidity and mortality. Interestingly, but not surprisingly, the inferior caval vein saturation had more predictive value with respect to morbidity and mortality. This is likely due to cerebral autoregulation which allows the superior caval vein oxygen saturation to drop less than the inferior caval vein oxygen saturation during the early stages of clinical deterioration. This goes against widely accepted dogma that superior caval vein oxygen saturations have more clinical utility than inferior caval vein oxygen saturations and the dogma held by some that inferior caval vein saturations have no clinical utility.

Additionally, there is value in regional monitoring of the adequacy of oxygen delivery to help identify regional morbidity. For instance, cerebral stroke, acute kidney injury, hepatic insufficiency, necrotizing enterocolitis, and limb ischemia may all be detected sooner with regional monitoring. Regional monitoring can be done by venous blood gases or by near infrared spectroscopy.

With respect to near infrared spectroscopy, critics will often discuss concerns regarding the accuracy of the estimate. When the cerebral near infrared spectroscopy value is compared to the internal jugular venous oxygen saturation or the superior caval vein oxygen saturation there may a 95% confidence interval of 10 to 15. The same holds true for renal near infrared spectroscopy and the inferior caval vein saturation. It must be kept in mind that the near infrared spectroscopy sensors are not over the same exact blood pool which is being sampled in these studies. Even the venous saturation in the same vein at the same site can differ between blood gas measurements due to streaming of blood.

The mass of blood changes based on the amount of oxygen in it. Particularly in venous blood, there can be variability of the amount of bound oxygen in small aliquots of blood as blood segregates geographically within the vessel based on mass and velocity. This phenomenon of streaming of venous blood-based oxygen saturation is particularly important in fetal circulation in which the inferior caval vein has both deoxygenated and oxygenated blood.

Due to the differences in mass, oxygenated blood and deoxygenated blood have different velocities and flow in different portions of the same vessel. In the fetal inferior caval vein the more oxygenated blood flows faster and segregates to the posterior aspect of the inferior caval vein. It ultimately enters the right atrium where the posteriorly placed Eustachian valve directs more of this oxygenated blood across the patent oval fossa and to the left side of the heart to encourage more oxygenated blood to enter the coronary and cerebral circulations.

Despite a clinically wide 95% confidence interval in the agreement between regional near infrared spectroscopy and regional venous saturation the correlation has been demonstrated to be quite good. This indicates that regional near infrared spectroscopy values hold significant trending value. An increasing near infrared spectroscopy value is predictive of an increasing venous saturation. Conversely, a decreasing near infrared spectroscopy values is predictive of a decreasing venous saturation.

Additionally, absolute values of near infrared spectroscopy monitoring have been demonstrated to be associated with risk of morbidity and mortality, irrespective of their absolute correlation with the underlying venous saturation.

Index	What Increases It	What Decreases It	Clinical Pitfall
A–V O_2 difference	↓ CO, ↑ VO_2	↑ CO, ↓ VO_2	May miss regional ischemia
Oxygen Extraction	Hypoxemia, anemia, tachycardia	Transfusion, FiO_2, sedation	Can be misleading in distributive shock
Venous Sat	↑ CO, ↓ VO_2	↓ CO, ↑ VO_2	Spuriously high in frank organ failure

Hemoglobin

As hemoglobin is what ultimately binds to oxygen and physically transports oxygen, monitoring the hemoglobin level is of clinical importance. Hemoglobin is a component of the oxygen content, cardiac output, and oxygen delivery equations. Hemoglobin can be quantified by blood analysis. Blood gas analysis can also provide an estimate of the hemoglobin.

There is no discrete threshold for a hemoglobin target in general. As with anything if there is evidence of inadequate oxygen delivery then a transfusion of packed red blood cells may help augment the venous oxygen saturation and improve the adequacy of oxygen delivery. There is a growing body of data that demonstrates packed red blood cell transfusions increase the venous oxygen saturation and help improve the arteriovenous oxygen saturation difference and oxygen extraction. The magnitude of improvement in the adequacy of oxygen delivery varies by circulatory physiology and the largest benefit seems to be in functionally univentricular multidistributive physiology. Two separate studies have demonstrated that there is improvement in the adequacy of oxygen delivery after a 15 ml/kg packed red blood cell transfusion in functionally univentricular multidistributive physiology when the pretransfusion hemoglobin is less than 12.5 mg/dl. This is not to say that a transfusion is required whenever the hemoglobin gets below this threshold but rather if there is inadequate systemic oxygen delivery and the hemoglobin is below this threshold.

Heart rate and rhythm

Heart rate and rhythm are routinely monitored. Heart rate is a component of the La Farge equation to estimate oxygen consumption and is a component of cardiac output as well. Heart rate can be quantified by palpating a pulse, cardiac auscultation, an arterial line waveform, pulse oximetry waveform, or electrocardiography. The rhythm can be interrogated by any of these as well although electrocardiography offers the most complete method for assessment of cardiac rhythm.

With regards to rate, there is no specific cutoff. Bradycardia can lead to impairment in cardiac output if stroke volume doesn't offset the decrease in heart rate while tachycardia can lead to impairment in cardiac output, particularly, if there is subsequent loss of atrioventricular synchrony. Within the oximetric framework, the effect of heart rate can be assessed by the oximetric indices already discussed whether it be arteriovenous oxygen saturation difference or oxygen extraction. If there is inadequacy of oxygen delivery and heart rate is believed to be contributing, then medical interventions to increase or decrease heart rate can be utilized or electrical pacing can also be utilized. The effects of these can then be monitored by the very same oximetric indices that first led to concern.

Arterial blood pressure

Arterial blood pressure is currently often at the forefront of clinical decision making. When viewed at from an oximetric standpoint arterial blood pressure is not in the oxygen content, cardiac output, or oxygen delivery equations. Arterial blood pressure is in the equation for systemic vascular resistance, however, which can indirectly influence cardiac output and oxygen delivery.

Arterial blood pressure can be monitored invasively using an arterial line and noninvasively using a blood pressure cuff. Arterial line blood pressure is advantageous as it allows for continuous monitoring of blood pressure. Additionally, arterial lines can allow for monitoring of the arterial waveform. The area under the curve of the arterial waveform can be used to quantify stroke volume. Variability in arterial line waveforms can also indicate intravascular hypovolemia or upper airway obstruction. Arterial lines, however, can be difficult to place and can lead to vascular injury, particularly in smaller children. Arterial lines may also produce spurious readings if the tip is in close proximity to the vessel wall. Blood pressure cuffs are advantageous as they are noninvasive, generally readily available, and are easy to use. Disadvantages of blood pressure cuffs are that improper size selection can lead to inaccurate readings. Both invasive and noninvasive strategies are limited in their accuracy with regard to diastolic blood pressure.

When considering any pressure, it is important to remember that pressure is the product of flow and resistance, and arterial blood pressure is thus the product of systemic blood flow and systemic vascular resistance. As discussed before, this highlights why arterial blood pressure cannot be considered to be reflective of systemic blood flow unless underlying changes in systemic vascular resistance are understood. If systemic vascular resistance is constant, then changes in blood pressure are directly reflective of changes in systemic blood flow. This has been demonstrated in patients with congenitally malformed hearts who undergo cardiac surgery and receive phenoxybenzamine for alpha-blockade, postoperatively.

Central venous pressure

Central venous pressure is often monitored in the pediatric cardiac intensive care unit. When viewed from an oximetric standpoint central venous pressure is not in the oxygen content, cardiac output, or oxygen delivery equations. Central venous pressure is in the equation for systemic vascular resistance, however, which can indirectly influence cardiac output and oxygen delivery.

Central venous pressure can only be monitored using invasive central lines. While monitoring central venous pressure can be clinically advantageous there might be difficulty with central line placement and line associated vascular injury.

When considering any pressure, it is important to remember that pressure is the product of flow and resistance, and central venous pressure is thus the product of venous blood flow and venous resistance. Central venous pressure is not equal to preload which is actually a loading force on the myocytes at end diastole. Equating the two offers no clinical advantage. And neither central venous pressure nor preload are equal to venous return which is a volume. Equating central venous pressure and venous flow is scientifically not sound since central venous pressure is also modulated by venous resistance and there is no routine monitoring of venous resistance. Venous flow (venous return) can decrease despite an increase in central venous pressure if there is an increase in venous resistance of greater magnitude.

Pulmonary artery pressure

Pulmonary artery pressure is not routinely monitored in the pediatric cardiac intensive care unit. When viewed from an oximetric standpoint, pulmonary artery pressure is not in the oxygen content, cardiac output, or oxygen delivery equations. Pulmonary artery pressure is in the equation for pulmonary vascular resistance, however, which can indirectly influence cardiac output and oxygen delivery.

Pulmonary artery pressure can only be monitored using invasive lines. While monitoring pulmonary artery pressure can be clinically advantageous there might be difficulty with pulmonary artery line placement and line associated vascular injury. Pulmonary artery catheter placement in pediatric patients can be more difficult than other venous lines. Smaller catheters may not be readily available for smaller patients.

When considering any pressure, it is important to remember that pressure is the product of flow and resistance and pulmonary artery pressure is thus the product of pulmonary arterial flow and pulmonary arterial vascular resistance.

Serum lactate

Serum lactate is often monitored, particularly in the postoperative pediatric cardiac patient. Lactate is produced by both aerobic and anaerobic mechanisms in the body. Aerobic mechanisms include aerobic glycolysis (Warburg effect), brain lactate shuttle, catecholamine-stimulated production, and fatty acid derivation. Anaerobic mechanisms include anaerobic glycolysis and obligate anaerobic metabolism. The most prevalent of these mechanics is generally anaerobic metabolism but that does not mean that in specific clinical settings the other mechanisms cannot become more prevalent.

While details of these mechanisms are beyond the scope of this text, a list of these mechanisms is presented to serve as a reminder that lactate is not simply a result of anaerobic metabolism. Assuming all increases in lactate are due to inadequate oxygen delivery is not accurate. This is also reinforced by the fact that lactate has several roles in the body and isn't simply a byproduct of anaerobic metabolism. Lactate can be shuttled to various tissues as a substrate for energy production in times of increased demand and is used as a cellular signaling molecule. As a signaling molecule, lactate helps regulate mitochondrial function, promotes angiogenesis, promotes erythropoiesis, promotes insulin secretion, promotes catecholamine release, inhibits cytotoxic T-cell activity, and promotes nitric oxide mediated vasodilation among other effects.

A detailed understanding of lactate should lead to an appreciation of its complexity and importance in the body which isn't simply isolated to anaerobic metabolism. In fact, studies have demonstrated that after pediatric cardiac surgery, serum lactate has poor correlation with oxygen delivery as quantified by oximetric indices. Serum lactate has been demonstrated to be more closely associated with serum glucose levels in the postoperative period. Increased glucose levels lead to increased glycolysis. Pyruvate is created during glycolysis and if the mitochondrial capacity to process pyruvate is exceeded then accumulating pyruvate is converted to lactate. The glucose level at which this occurs is different from patient to patient and even from time to time in the same patient.

Clinically, this means that lactate levels need to be interpreted with caution. If lactate levels are high but oximetric indices indicate adequate oxygen delivery, then the lactate should not be interpreted to be indicative of inadequate oxygen delivery. While this seems obvious, it is important to highlight this as a reminder that the arteriovenous oxygen saturation difference and oxygen extraction are both direct markers of oxygen delivery while lactate is an indirect marker.

Additionally, the oft-cited and oft-used cutoff of 2 mmol/L is an arbitrary cutoff. Studies demonstrating lactate levels predictive of morbidity and mortality identify a cutoff between 4 and 5 mmol/L. What seems to have most prognostic utility, specifically in patients with distributive shock and/or receiving mechanical circulatory support is the change in lactate levels over time. Increases of 0.5 mmol/L/hr should attract attention and trigger review of oximetric indices. Clearance of less than 0.5 mmol/L/hr while receiving mechanical circulatory support should attract attention and may indicate inadequate support.

Some have proposed combined oximetric and lactate metrics. Specifically, there is a venous saturation to lactate ratio. This has been shown to have greater prognostic utility than an isolated lactate level. With the aforementioned discussion the reason for this should be relatively intuitive and supports the above comments on lactate and its clinical utility.

Lactate is measured with serum analysis using blood. Either arterial or venous blood can be utilized for this. Lactate levels are often included in point of care blood gas analyses.

Partial pressure of carbon dioxide

Partial pressure of carbon dioxide is often monitored in the cardiac intensive care unit. Monitoring the partial pressure of carbon dioxide is important to help titrate ventilatory support, particularly invasive mechanical ventilation. Partial pressure of carbon dioxide can be directly quantified by blood gas analysis. The partial pressure of carbon dioxide can be quantified in any circulation whether it be arterial, capillary, or venous blood. One must be mindful of where the blood was sampled from to understand how to best interpret the results.

Variable	Direct Measure	Indirect / Estimate	Advantages	Limitations
Arterial Sat	Blood gas	Pulse oximetry	Accurate / Noninvasive	Invasive draw / less accurate in hypoxemia
Venous Sat	Venous gas	NIRS	Accurate / Noninvasive & continuous	Requires line / sensor cost
Hemoglobin	Blood analysis	Blood gas estimate	Objective	Invasive, intermittent
CO_2	Blood gas	End-tidal CO_2	Direct / Continuous	Sampling site variability
Blood Pressure	Arterial line / cuff	Waveform analysis	Continuous /noninvasive	Not equal to flow
Lactate	Serum analysis	None	Prognostic trends	Not always delivery-linked

Metric	"Concerning" Range	Prognostic Notes
A–V O_2 diff	>30–40%	↑ morbidity, mortality
O_2 extraction	>30–40%	↑ morbidity, mortality
Lactate	>4–5 mmol/L	Trend/change more valuable
NIRS (cerebral/renal)	Falling trend	Strong predictive value

While normative ranges exist for the partial pressure of carbon dioxide (approximately 35 to 45 mmHg in arterial blood) the partial pressure of carbon dioxide must be interpreted with respect to the overall acid-base status as well as the serial change over time. A patient with a 60-mmHg partial pressure of carbon dioxide, pH of 7.40, no respiratory distress, and a serum bicarbonate level of 30 may not require escalation in ventilatory support while a patient with a 50-mmHg partial pressure of carbon dioxide, pH of 7.30, severe respiratory distress, and a serum bicarbonate level of 18 may require escalation in ventilatory support.

What this highlights is that changes in the partial pressure of carbon dioxide may be due to several reasons. An elevated partial pressure of carbon dioxide may be secondary to inadequate ventilation due to respiratory muscle weakness, airway obstruction, or parenchymal dysfunction. It may also be in response to a metabolic alkalosis which may be secondary to ingestion or intravascular hypovolemia. The clinical interpretation and response to the resulting value will differ based on the overall clinical status and the circumstances felt to be surrounding perturbations.

It should be noted that the partial pressure of carbon dioxide is higher in the venous rather than arterial blood. This difference is generally less than 10 mmHg. An elevated veno-arterial carbon dioxide difference may be secondary to decreased cardiac output.

End tidal carbon dioxide monitoring by blood gas analysis

End tidal carbon dioxide monitoring can be a helpful adjunct to monitoring the partial pressure of carbon dioxide by blood gas analysis. End tidal carbon dioxide monitoring utilizes a sensor that is placed in-line with a respiratory support device. At the moment, such end tidal carbon dioxide devices are available for conventional nasal cannula or invasive endotracheal tubes.

These devices utilize infrared spectroscopy to detect exhaled carbon dioxide and can quantify the amount of carbon dioxide in the exhaled blood. This value can be continuously monitored without requiring a blood gas to be drawn and analyzed. The benefit is that this provides continuous estimation of the partial pressure of carbon dioxide without continuous blood gases. There are not many disadvantages of end tidal carbon dioxide monitoring although it does introduce some additional dead space into the respiratory circuit. Mainstream capnography in which the device is attached to the airway tubing itself can add 5 to 15 ml of dead space while sidestream capnography devices add less than 1 ml of dead space. The introduced deadspace may be of greater issue in critically ill neonates and infants compared to larger children or young adults.

End tidal carbon dioxide monitoring provides an estimated partial pressure of carbon dioxide but also provides a waveform. This waveform plots partial pressure of carbon dioxide over time. Various patterns in this waveform can indicate different clinical occurrences such as the "shark fin" appearance (distinctive upward slope in the third phase of the waveform) which is usually due to airway obstruction. Thus, recognition of various waveform shapes can be clinically useful.

The estimated partial pressure of carbon dioxide must be interpreted with understanding of what may affect the values and the relationship of this value to the underlying arterial partial pressure of carbon dioxide. Generally, the gradient between the arterial and end tidal partial pressure of carbon dioxide is less than 10. A larger gradient could be secondary to decreased cardiac output as with the veno-arterial carbon dioxide difference. But an elevation may also be secondary to a large leak around the respiratory support circuit or leak due to an open mouth.

It is important to note that just because there may be a large arterial to end tidal carbon dioxide difference that this does not mean that the end tidal carbon dioxide monitoring is not helpful. In fact, quite to the contrary, it may be a helpful monitoring tool to indicate a worsening airway leak or worsening cardiac output. Even despite an absolute difference between the two, the relative difference may stay the same and still allow for reasonable estimation of the arterial partial pressure of carbon dioxide and help minimize the need for blood gas analysis to adjust respiratory support.

End organ function

End organ function is routinely monitored in the pediatric cardiac intensive care unit. As this is fairly prevalent it will not be covered at length in this text. Nonetheless, laboratory evaluation of end organ function is important as it helps identify at what point oxygen delivery truly is becoming inadequate for specific organs.

With respect to the heart, brain natriuretic peptide, troponin, and creatinine kinase MB may be utilized to help evaluate cardiac function. Of course, heart function with regards to pump function is best assessed by echocardiography.

With respect to the kidneys, serum creatinine as well as cystatin C may be utilized to help evaluate kidney function. Classification systems of acute kidney injury utilize serum creatinine and thus creatinine is of particular importance. It is important to keep in mind that urine output is also a metric of kidney function.

With respect to the liver, aspartate aminotransferase, alanine aminotransferase levels, alkaline phosphatase, gamma-glutamyl transferase, bilirubin, albumin, prothrombin time, and international normalized ratio may be utilized to help evaluate hepatic function.

Electrolyte levels

Electrolyte levels are frequently monitored. Electrolyte levels can be ordered in various combinations and be assessed by serum blood collection. Additionally, some electrolyte levels are included in blood gas analyses.

Trends in electrolyte levels are likely more telling than absolute values. Electrolyte levels will often be deranged in clinically ill children but stable levels or changes over time may lead to less adverse events than acute changes. While unit-adopted electrolyte levels are present in many pediatric cardiac intensive care units and are helpful in automating electrolyte repletion, it should be noted that electrolyte levels may need to be tailored for specific patients and specific clinical settings.

Additional cardiac output and vascular resistance monitoring

There is an increasing number of devices that aim to noninvasively estimate cardiac output and systemic vascular resistance. These devices utilize various methods including, but not limited to, electrical impedance and pulse wave analysis. These devices are improving in accuracy as the technology and algorithms that underpin them are improving.

If real-time cardiac output monitoring is being utilized, whether this be by thermodilution, impedance, or pulse wave analysis, it is important to understand that cardiac output simply quantifies the cardiac output and does not account for all of oxygen delivery. Thus, it should not be used in lieu of oximetric indices but as a component of them.

Physiologic data streaming

Physiologic data streaming platforms are now becoming more widely adopted. These platforms integrate data and waveforms from various monitoring devices allowing for centralized collection and storage of data. The data are collected with high temporal resolution. These platforms do require thoughtful implementation to ensure regulatory compliance and reliable data storage. But such platforms allow for centralized, often even remote, viewing of multiple data streams in a user-friendly, user-defined layout. The raw data can also be utilized to perform calculations in real-time, utilize machine learning and artificial intelligence to help develop/validate/deploy algorithms, or refine alarms. These features allow for increased efficiency of monitoring strategies.

4
Medical and procedural interventions

The aim of this textbook is to be concise and incorporate fundamental elements of pediatric cardiac intensive care within the oximetric framework. As such, the goal of this chapter is not to go into detail of every medical and procedural intervention in the pediatric cardiac intensive care unit but to cover how to conceptualize them in the oximetric framework.

Medical interventions

A number of medications are used in the pediatric cardiac intensive care unit. This section will cover medications by class, understanding that not all medications within a class will have the same magnitude of effect on the various domains of oxygen delivery. Detailed nuances of each medication lie outside the scope of this textbook and could require an entire textbook in and of itself.

Inotropes are frequently used in the pediatric cardiac intensive care unit. These include, but are not limited to, epinephrine, norepinephrine, dopamine, dobutamine, milrinone, levosimendan, isoproterenol, and calcium. Inotropes increase contractility which helps increase stroke volume, which increases cardiac output. Various agents have different mechanisms and different secondary effects. Some of these will be covered in other sections. Some of these agents will increase myocardial oxygen consumption, while others may cause vasoconstriction, and others may cause vasodilation.

Inodilators are medications that are inotropes and vasodilators. These include dobutamine, milrinone, levosimendan, and isoproterenol. Inodilators are particularly impactful since they affect multiple components of oxygen delivery in a beneficial way. Stroke volume is augmented by an increase in contractility as well as decrease in afterload. This increase in stroke volume results in an increase in cardiac output barring other changes. The inotropic and vasodilatory effects may have differing magnitudes at varying doses of the same inodilator. Thus, these medications must be titrated with this in mind.

Inoconstrictors are medications that are inotropes and vasoconstrictors. These include epinephrine, norepinephrine, and dopamine. Inotropy, or the augmentation of contractility, increases stroke volume. Vasoconstriction, however, increases afterload which can lead to a decrease in stroke volume. At different doses of the same inoconstrictor, the inotropic effects and vasoconstrictive effects may be different. Thus, these agents must be titrated with this in mind.

A purer inotrope is calcium. Whether administered as a bolus or infusion, calcium has been associated with increased contractility, increased venous saturation, and decreased oxygen extraction.

Vasoconstrictors are medications that simply constrict the blood vessels. These include vasopressin and phenylephrine. These medications simply increase afterload without an increase in inotropy. In the setting of the oximetric framework, the utility of pure vasoconstrictors certainly comes into question. Previous chapters have discussed that arterial blood pressure and oxygen delivery are not positively correlated. If arterial blood pressure is being augmented due to an increase in systemic vascular resistance and not because of systemic blood flow, then it is more likely that oxygen delivery will become less adequate. This occurs as an increase in afterload may lead to a decrease in stroke volume. With a pure vasoconstrictor effect, vasopressin and phenylephrine are unlikely to directly improve oxygen delivery despite increases in blood pressure. This has been demonstrated to be the case in patients in the pediatric cardiac intensive care unit with functionally univentricular physiologies or biventricular physiology. There are some neurohormonal effects of vasopressin, in particular, that may make it beneficial in some situations, specifically related to patients with capillary leak but there are minimal data regarding this at the moment.

Vasodilators are medications that dilate the blood vessels and help reduce systemic vascular resistance and afterload. These include nicardipine, sodium nitroprusside, clevidipine, and hydralazine. While other medications also cause vasodilation, they also have other effects and have been discussed elsewhere. Stroke volume increases as afterload decreases, thus leading to improving oxygen delivery. It is worth noting that there are no objective data to demonstrate that use of nicardipine in neonatal patients leads to a decrease in inotropy. Data regarding use of nicardipine in neonates demonstrates that there is no associated decrease in serum calcium levels, no direct decrease in contractility, and no negative effect on oxygen delivery.

Alpha blocking agents, such as phenoxybenzamine and phentolamine, decrease systemic vascular resistance, and thus, afterload. Both have been associated with improved adequacy of oxygen delivery.

Chronotropes are medications that increase heart rate. These include epinephrine, norepinephrine, dopamine, dobutamine, isoproterenol, atropine, and xanthine derivatives (theophylline, aminophylline, caffeine). These medications have various mechanisms and have varying other effects. These must be kept in mind when trying to select an agent for chronotropic effect. As discussed previously, cardiac output is the product of heart rate and stroke volume so if heart rate increases without a decrease in stroke volume of greater magnitude, then increasing heart rate should lead to an increase in stroke volume.

Related to chronotropes is electrical pacing. If pacemaker wires are present, then heart rate can be augmented by pacing. The impact on oxygen delivery is the same as discussed with chronotropes.

There is, theoretically, a point at which additional increases in heart rate could impair stroke volume by decreasing diastolic filling time and, thus, ventricular preload. There are not great data to objectively identify when this phenomenon occurs. It is also likely patient- and setting-specific.

Beta-blockers are utilized for arrhythmia as well as heart failure. There are a variety of beta-blockers which have variable effects on subtypes of beta-receptors as well as other receptor types. With respect to the components of oxygen delivery, beta-blockers have no effect on oxygen content, decrease heart rate, have no direct effect on preload, may reduce afterload, and may decrease contractility. It is important to note that if a beta-blocker is being utilized as an anti-arrhythmic and there is lack of atrioventricular synchrony when starting the beta-blocker, that restoration of atrioventricular synchrony may also lead to an increase in stroke volume. Depending on the specific beta-blocker utilized and the dose utilized, there may be various magnitudes of effects on the individual components of oxygen delivery. Based on the relative magnitude of these effects, the adequacy of oxygen delivery may get better or worse. Thus, it is important to closely monitor oximetric indices when initiating a beta-blocker.

Other medications are also utilized for anti-arrhythmic effects. One such commonly utilized medication is amiodarone. Amiodarone has been associated with hemodynamic collapse and cardiac arrest in pediatric intensive care unit patients. Data have demonstrated that this effect is due to direct effects of amiodarone which can decrease myocardial contractility but that this effect may also be due to the solvent in amiodarone and/or the rate of infusion of intravenous amiodarone. Nonetheless, amiodarone may decrease contractility and thus lead to a decrease in stroke volume, cardiac output, and oxygen delivery. Other agents such as digoxin, procainamide, or intravenous sotalol may not have such negative effects.

Analgesia and anesthetic medications such as opiates, benzodiazepines, dexmedetomidine, clonidine, phenobarbital, ketamine, and propofol can help decrease oxygen extraction, improving the adequacy of oxygen delivery. Various agents can have other effects, namely vasodilation, and thus the specifics regarding each agent must be considered when selecting a specific agent. Muscle relaxants, or paralytic medications further help decrease oxygen extraction.

Procedural interventions

A number of procedural interventions may occur in the pediatric cardiac intensive care unit. These can also impact oxygen delivery. As with the medical interventions this section is not meant to be a definitive guide to such procedures but is simply

Class	Examples	Primary Effect on O_2 Delivery	Other Key Effects
Inotropes	Epinephrine, Dopamine, Milrinone	↑ Contractility → ↑ SV, ↑ CO	Some ↑ VO_2 (myocardial)
Inodilators	Dobutamine, Milrinone	↑ Contractility & ↓ Afterload → ↑ SV, ↑ CO	Vasodilation at higher doses
Inoconstrictors	Epinephrine, Norepinephrine	↑ Contractility (↑ SV) + ↑ Afterload (↓ SV)	Dose-dependent balance
Vasoconstrictors	Vasopressin, Phenylephrine	↑ Afterload → ↓ SV, ↓ CO	↑ BP without ↑ DO_2
Vasodilators	Nicardipine, SNP	↓ Afterload → ↑ SV, ↑ CO	No direct contractility effect
Chronotropes	Isoproterenol, Atropine	↑ HR → ↑ CO (if SV preserved)	At high HR may ↓ preload
Beta-blockers	Propranolol, Metoprolol	↓ HR, ↓ Contractility	Restore AV synchrony may ↑ SV
Anti-arrhythmics	Amiodarone	↓ Contractility → ↓ SV, ↓ CO	Risk of collapse if rapid infusion
Sedatives/Analgesics	Opiates, Benzos, Dexmedetomidine	↓ VO_2 (↓ extraction)	Some vasodilation
Paralytics	Rocuronium, Vecuronium	↓ VO_2 (↓ extraction)	Facilitate ventilation

meant to frame how procedural interventions may impact the adequacy of oxygen delivery. Thus, the specifics on the techniques and methods of procedures will not be covered here.

Venous line insertion is one of the most frequent procedural interventions in the pediatric cardiac intensive care unit. This does not necessarily directly impact the adequacy of oxygen delivery but does help facilitate the assessment of it by allowing for the quantification of venous oxygen saturation.

Arterial line insertion is also done in the pediatric cardiac intensive care unit. Similar to venous line insertion, this does not directly impact the adequacy of oxygen delivery but does help facilitate the assessment of it by allowing for the quantification of arterial oxygen saturation.

Chest tube insertion can help drain the pleural space of fluid or evacuate it of air. Pleural effusions can negatively impact respiratory mechanics and lead to impairment of oxygenation and ventilation. Successful chest tube insertion and drainage of pleural effusions can lead to improvement in oxygenation and thus can help improve oxygen content which can then help improve oxygen delivery. Successful chest tube insertion and evacuation of a pneumothorax can also lead to improvement in oxygenation and thus can help improve oxygen content which can then help improve oxygen delivery. Significant pleural effusion, hemothorax, or pneumothorax can also lead to a reduction in stroke volume and thus cardiac output. Chest tube insertion can thus help improve stroke volume and cardiac output in these settings as well.

Similarly to chest tube insertion, pericardial drain placement can help drain fluid from around the heart.

Pericardial fluid may be serous, infectious, or sanguineous and any type of fluid can lead to

Procedure	Mechanism	Effect on O_2 Delivery
Venous line	Access for SvO_2 monitoring	Facilitates assessment
Arterial line	Access for SaO_2, ABP	Facilitates assessment
Chest tube	Removes air/fluid → improves ventilation & stroke volume	↑ O_2 content & ↑ CO
Pericardial drain	Relieves tamponade → improves SV	↑ CO
Intubation	Stabilizes ventilation/oxygenation	To be detailed in respiratory chapter

tamponade which leads to a reduction in stroke volume and thus cardiac output.

Intubation and extubation are also relatively common procedures in the cardiac intensive care unit but the physiologic effects of these will be discussed in a dedicated chapter.

5
Cardiopulmonary bypass and its effects

The goal of this chapter is not to go into detail regarding the deployment of cardiopulmonary bypass and all its effects but to cover how to conceptualize cardiopulmonary bypass in the oximetric framework and how its effects may impact the components of oxygen delivery and the adequacy of oxygen delivery. It is assumed that the reader understands the basic concepts of cardiopulmonary bypass.

Cardiopulmonary bypass helps facilitate cardiac surgery, allowing the surgeons to operate on a non-beating heart while ensuring the organs get adequate oxygen delivery. The details of the circuit will not be discussed here but, in brief, the cardiopulmonary bypass circuit consists of a venous limb, oxygenator, pump, and an arterial limb. The venous limb facilitates gathering venous blood and bringing it to the oxygenator and pump which facilitate gas exchange and propulsion of the blood. The arterial limb then helps gets the oxygenated blood back into the body so it can get to the organs.

The issues surrounding cardiopulmonary bypass surround the inflammatory processes triggered by the circuit as well as the need to ensure that cardiopulmonary bypass is facilitating enough oxygen delivery from a technical oxygenator and pump standpoint.

Inflammatory effects of cardiopulmonary bypass effect

As blood exits the body and courses through the cardiopulmonary bypass circuit it is exposed to human-made materials. These non-endothelial surfaces of the circuit trigger activation of the complement system, activation of the coagulation cascade, and increase of platelet activation. This inflammatory response usually peaks within the first 48 hours after bypass. The degree and duration of response can impact morbidity and mortality.

Inflammation can have a few overarching effects through which oxygen delivery may be impacted, including an increase in metabolic rate, mitochondrial dysfunction, decrease in contractility, and shivering.

Metabolic rate increases with inflammation for several reasons. One of these is cellular activation. When activated, neutrophils, macrophages, and platelets all consume more oxygen to help facilitate phagocytosis, generation of reactive oxygen species, and cytokine synthesis among other tasks. Reduction of the inflammatory response and cellular activation may be modifiable by minimizing circuit length, minimizing circuit surface area, utilizing biocompatible coatings in the circuit, and utilizing modified ultrafiltration. Pharmacologic interventions that have been explored to help minimize circuit related inflammation include corticosteroids, tranexamic acid, aprotinin, and dexmedetomidine. There are conflicting data regarding corticosteroids and clinical outcome, with most data indicating corticosteroids have minimal clinical benefit if any. Tranexamic acid is generally used, clinically, as an antifibrinolytic to reduce bleeding although it may reduce inflammatory mediators. Aprotinin has been demonstrated to reduce cytokine response in children although its clinical use decreased due to data from the adult population regarding its renal effects. There are increasing data now to demonstrate that dexmedetomidine can help reduce the inflammatory response.

Mitochondrial dysfunction can occur because of disruption of mitochondrial oxidative phosphorylation. This disruption in mitochondrial oxidative phosphorylation is generally secondary to reactive oxygen species and cytokines and results in less efficient adenosine triphosphate production. This efficiency in adenosine triphosphate production refers to the amount of adenosine triphosphate produced per amount of oxygen, thus in the setting of mitochondrial dysfunction, more oxygen may be necessary to produce the same amount of adenosine triphosphate compared to the normal state. This can often clinically manifest as a lactatemia in the setting of adequate systemic oxygen delivery. Maintaining oxygen content, maintaining normothermia, avoiding rapid rewarming, avoiding acidemia, and minimizing beta-agonism can help the mitochondria recover more efficient function. There are increasing data, albeit much of it adult, regarding thiamine, ascorbic acid, carnitine, methylene blue, and N-acetylcysteine to help improve mitochondrial function.

Myocardial function and contractility may be negatively impacted by bypass. Tumor necrosis factor alpha and interleukin-1B levels both increase after bypass and both can lead to decreased cardiac contractility. Additionally, myocardial edema may occur due to inflammation-induced capillary leak. This myocardial edema can lead to myocardial stiffening and impair contractility. Both mechanisms lead to a decrease in stroke volume and, thus, cardiac output.

Shivering can occur due to inflammation as well as the thermoregulatory effects of cardiopulmonary bypass. While it may seem odd to mention this in such a text, it is an important consideration as the increase in oxygen consumption with shivering can be significant, particularly in neonates and infants. Shivering can be controlled by maintaining normothermia and maintaining adequate levels of sedation and pain control.

Effect	**Mechanism**	**Impact on Oxygen Delivery (DO_2/VO_2 balance)**	**Mitigation Strategies**
↑ Metabolic rate	Immune cell activation	↑ VO_2	Circuit coatings, ultrafiltration, pharmacologics
Mitochondrial dysfunction	ROS, cytokines	↓ ATP/O_2 efficiency	Normothermia, avoid rapid rewarming, antioxidants
↓ Contractility	TNF-α, IL-1β, edema	↓ SV → ↓ CO → ↓ DO_2	Anti-inflammatory agents, inotropes
Shivering	Thermoregulation	↑ VO_2	Sedation, analgesia, warming

Modulation of oxygen delivery via the cardiopulmonary bypass circuit

Careful titration of various parameters is necessary while on cardiopulmonary bypass. While on cardiopulmonary bypass with cardioplegia in the operating room, the native heart is void of most preload, has no contractility, and experiences relatively high afterload. These conditions have implications for when separating from bypass; but, while on bypass, the circuit is responsible for circulation and oxygen delivery.

The physiologic principles and considerations remain the same. The circuit requires preload to continue functioning and this circulatory volume dictates what the pump's output or stroke volume can be. The pump must also overcome afterload and increasing afterload will require more pump effort to circulate the same amount of volume. Pump revolutions become the correlate of heart rate and contractility. Thus, volume status and pump revolutions per minute are important to modulate. Additionally, oxygen content is intuitively monitored while on bypass and augmentation of the fraction of inspired oxygen and hemoglobin can help augment oxygen content and thus oxygen delivery.

Monitoring oxygen delivery and its adequacy does not differ from previously discussed. Venous saturations or near infrared spectroscopy have been demonstrated to be helpful. Multi-site near infrared spectroscopy can be particularly helpful as it can help lend insights into the adequacy of oxygen delivery to different regions, allowing for regional issues to be identified. Monitoring pump flow in isolation is not adequate as monitoring delivery in isolation of consumption does not allow for assessment of the adequacy of oxygen delivery.

Circuit Parameter	**Physiologic Analog**	**Oximetric Effect**
Venous reservoir volume	Preload	Dictates pump stroke volume
Pump RPM	Contractility	Higher RPM → ↑ flow/CO
Afterload (arterial resistance)	Systemic vascular resistance	Higher afterload → ↓ pump output
FiO_2 + Hb	Oxygen content	Directly ↑ DO_2

6
Circulatory physiologies

When discussing patients in the cardiac intensive care unit it is easy to get lost in the various anatomic labels. But care for patients in the cardiac intensive care unit is more dependent on the circulatory physiology rather than the specific anatomy. Several different anatomies may result in the same circulatory physiology, and the same anatomy may result in a different circulatory physiology depending on the stage of palliation or repair; thus, it becomes easier to frame thought based on circulatory physiology rather than anatomy.

The next several chapters will discuss the hemodynamic considerations of various circulatory physiologies and discuss the nuances of the oximetric framework for each. While each circulatory physiology is covered separately it is important to note that there may be elements of multiple circulatory physiologies present in a single moment, and identification of the predominant one often will guide overall care.

For the sake of the text the following categories of circulatory physiologies will be utilized: fully septated biventricular circulation, left to right shunt, limitation to pulmonary blood flow, limitation to systemic blood flow, preoperative transposition, functionally univentricular, and heart failure. Some of these categories also certainly have meaningful subsets, specifically the functionally univentricular category.

Understanding of these circulatory physiologies is important as the oximetric framework does not change across the physiologies but rather the magnitude of effect and some of the interplay between components of oxygen delivery do.

Oximetric concepts important to keep in mind for each physiologic state, the relative pulmonary and systemic flows, what mediates cardiac output, and what mediates the arterial saturation.

7
Fully septated biventricular physiology

Fully septated biventricular physiology represents the normal situation. There are normal systemic venous connections, usually arranged atria, concordant atrioventricular connections, right-handed ventricular topology, concordant ventriculo-arterial connections, and spiraling great arteries.

Direction of blood flow

In fully septated biventricular physiology, systemic venous and coronary venous blood comes back to the right atrium. This blood then goes to the right ventricle, via the tricuspid valve, which pumps the blood to the lungs via the pulmonary trunk and the branch pulmonary arteries. The blood then gets oxygenated and returns to the left atrium via the pulmonary veins. This blood then enters the left ventricle, via the mitral valve, which pumps it to the head and body via the aorta.

Distribution of blood flow into the pulmonary and systemic circulations

In fully septated biventricular physiology all the blood pumped by the right ventricle goes to the pulmonary circulation and all the blood pumped by the left ventricle goes to the systemic circulation.

Because the pulmonary and systemic circulations are in series, there is the ability for independent regulation of pulmonary and systemic blood flow. Pulmonary and systemic blood flow must be relatively equal over time although in the short-term there may be slight differences based on bronchial and Thebesian venous return, transient retention of blood in compliant vascular bloods, or capillary leak. Significant imbalances in pulmonary and systemic blood flow in this circulation would lead to volume overload in various sites.

Saturations

Arterial saturation in this circulation is equal to the pulmonary venous saturation. The venous saturation will generally be within 35 of the arterial saturation. The pulmonary artery saturation will be a weighted average of the inferior caval vein, superior caval vein, and coronary sinus saturations.

Pressures and volumes

As this is the usual arrangement there are no special considerations for pressures and volumes.

Clinical considerations in the context of the oximetric framework

There are no particular special clinical considerations in the context of the oximetric framework as this is the normal situation and thus has been described in earlier discussions of the oximetric framework.

8
Left to right shunt physiology

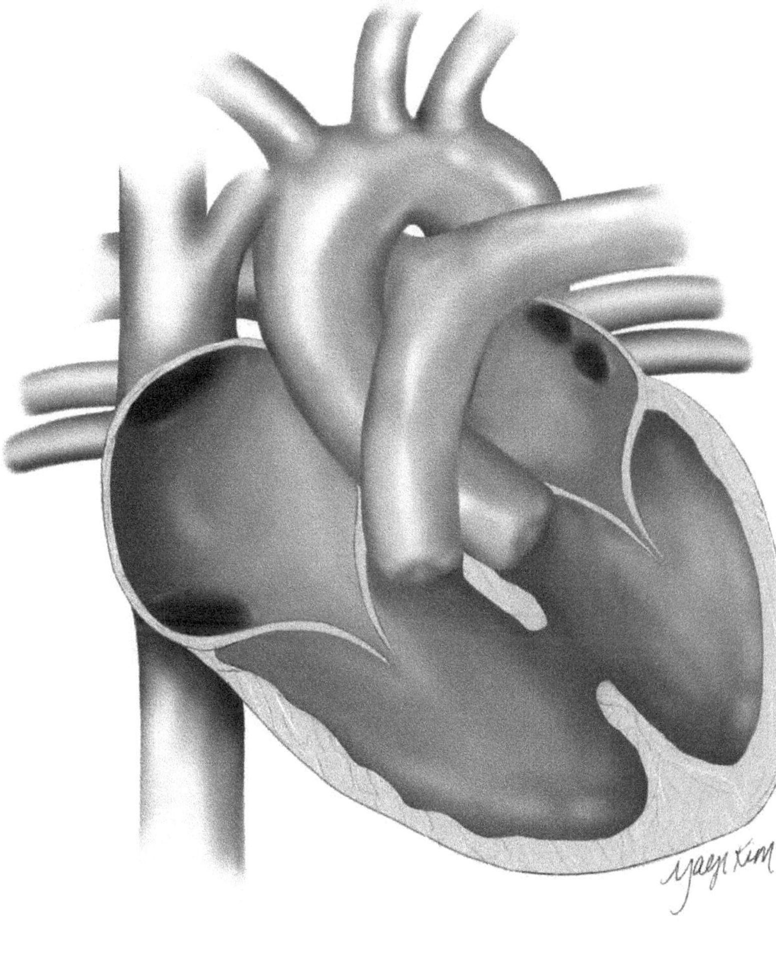

Left to right shunt physiology represents the situation in which blood from the left side of the heart shunts from the systemic circulation and mixes with blood in the right side of the heart. Thus, there is shunting of blood and mixing of blood pools with differing oxygen saturations as pulmonary venous blood and systemic venous blood mix.

A left to right shunt may result from intracardiac or extracardiac shunts. Intracardiac left to right shunts include an interatrial shunt (atrial septal defect, sinus venosus defect), ventricular septal defect, aortopulmonary window, patent arterial duct, surgically created systemic to pulmonary artery shunts, aortopulmonary collaterals, pulmonary arteriovenous malformations, and anomalous pulmonary venous connection.

Direction of blood flow

In the presence of a left to right shunt the systemic venous and coronary venous blood comes back to the right atrium. The blood then goes to the right ventricle which pumps it to the lungs via the pulmonary trunk and the branch pulmonary arteries. The blood then gets oxygenated and returns to the left atrium via the pulmonary veins. The blood then should enter the left ventricle which pumps this blood to the head and the body via the aorta.

However, depending on the level of the shunt, blood may not progress forward. If there is an atrial level shunt, some blood will leave the left atrium via the shunt and enter the right atrium. If there is a ventricular level shunt, some blood will leave the left ventricle via the shunt and enter the right ventricle. If there is an aortopulmonary window, some blood will leave the aorta via the shunt and enter the pulmonary trunk. If there is an arterial duct or surgical shunt, then some blood will leave the aorta via the shunt and enter the pulmonary trunk.

Distribution of blood flow into the pulmonary and systemic circulations

In left to right shunt physiology, all the blood returning to the right heart from the systemic veins and the coronary veins enters the pulmonary circulation. However, in addition to this, whatever blood comes from the left side of the heart to the right side via the left to right shunt also enters the pulmonary circulation. This means that the amount of pulmonary blood flow exceeds the amount of systemic blood flow.

Saturations

Arterial saturation in this circulation should be near 100% if there is no pulmonary venous desaturation, thus arterial saturation should be equal to the pulmonary vein saturation.

The systemic venous saturation will be dependent on several factors but if there is adequate systemic oxygen delivery (ratio of both delivery and consumption) then the systemic venous saturation should be within 35 of the arterial saturation.

Pulmonary artery saturation will not be equal to the systemic venous saturation due to the left to right shunt. Depending on the level of the shunt, there will be an increase in saturation when compared to the systemic veins. In the presence of an atrial septal defect this will occur at the level of the right atrium, in the presence of ventricular septal defect it will generally occur in the pulmonary trunk, and in the presence of an aortopulmonary window or surgical shunt it will generally occur in the pulmonary trunk or branch pulmonary arteries.

Pressures and volumes

In left to right shunt physiology there is an increase in pulmonary blood flow and a decrease in systemic blood flow. The relative volumes of this change with the ratio of pulmonary to systemic resistance. What chambers are volume loaded depends on the level of the shunt.

In the setting of an atrial level shunt, the right atrium, the right ventricle, and the pulmonary artery are volume loaded. In the setting of a ventricular level shunt, the pulmonary artery, the left atrium, and the left ventricle are volume loaded. In the setting of an arterial duct or aortopulmonary window the pulmonary artery, the left atrium, and the left ventricle are volume loaded. In the setting of a surgical systemic to pulmonary artery shunt the pulmonary artery, left atrium, and left ventricle are volume loaded.

In the setting of an atrial level shunt, the right atrium and right ventricle are pressure loaded. In the setting of a ventricular level shunt, the right ventricle, pulmonary trunk, left atrium, and left ventricle are pressure loaded. In the setting of an aortopulmonary window, arterial duct, or surgically placed systemic to pulmonary shunt, the pulmonary arteries, the left atrium, and the left ventricle are pressure loaded.

In the setting of a large ventricular septal defect, it is often stated that pressures between the two ventricles are “equal.” While mean pressures may be similar, the pressure relationship is not fixed throughout the cardiac cycle. Instead, there are instantaneous pressure gradients that vary as the ventricles contract

and relax, and as the atrioventricular and arterial valves open and close.
During early systole, when both ventricles are contracting but before the arterial valves open, left ventricular pressure rises more rapidly than right ventricular pressure, creating a transient left-to-right gradient. Once the aortic and pulmonary valves open, the pressures in the two ventricles converge more closely, but small oscillations remain depending on relative outflow impedance. In diastole, particularly in the setting of elevated right atrial pressure or tricuspid regurgitation, right-to-left gradients may briefly occur before mitral valve opening equilibrates the chambers.

Thus, shunting across a large ventricular septal defect is not unidirectional at every instant of the cardiac cycle. The direction of shunting varies with these changing pressure relationships. However, because systemic resistance is normally higher than pulmonary resistance, the integrated flow over time remains predominantly left-to-right. It is this net left-to-right shunt that drives the hemodynamic consequences of volume loading of the pulmonary circulation.

Clinical considerations in the context of the oximetric framework

In the setting of left to right shunts, a widening arteriovenous oxygen saturation difference or increasing oxygen extraction imply worsening adequacy of oxygen delivery. The primary reason for worsening adequacy of oxygen delivery is generally a decrease in cardiac output (systemic blood flow).

When the major components of oxygen delivery (oxygen extraction, oxygen content, heart rate, preload, afterload, contractility) are considered the special considerations in the setting come with respect to oxygen content, preload, and afterload.

Oxygen content is important but perhaps slightly indirectly. Blood transfusions have been demonstrated to be transiently advantageous in the setting of left to right shunts, specifically, ventricular level shunts. This is because of the increase in total cardiac output (rheologic effects), the increase in oxygen content, but as well as an increase in pulmonary vascular resistance which may help decrease the shunt fraction for at least a brief period of time.

Preload is important as increasing preload increases the total cardiac output including both pulmonary and systemic flow. If systemic oxygen delivery is believed to be inadequate, then systemic blood flow can be augmented by provided a fluid bolus which will increase both systemic and pulmonary blood flow.

Afterload is important as decreasing left ventricular afterload can increase systemic blood flow, particularly if this translates into a decrease in the systemic vascular resistance to pulmonary vascular resistance ratio. Reduction in afterload with vasodilators can thus be helpful. Often this consists of agents such as angiotensin converting enzyme inhibitors which can be utilized outpatient. Inpatient, however, milrinone can also be utilized. Milrinone can also improve contractility, further improving systemic oxygen delivery.

Surgical intervention or catheter-based intervention should be considered when medical management is unable to maintain systemic oxygen delivery.

Component	Role	Clinical Considerations
Oxygen content	Important (Hb transfusion may transiently improve DO_2, also ↑ PVR to reduce shunt)	Transfusion effects often temporary
Preload	↑ Preload ↑ total CO (systemic + pulmonary)	Fluids can help systemic DO_2
Afterload	↓ LV afterload → ↑ systemic flow	Vasodilators (ACEi, milrinone) helpful
Contractility	Inotropes may augment systemic flow	Milrinone helpful (dual effect)

9
Limitation to pulmonary blood flow physiology

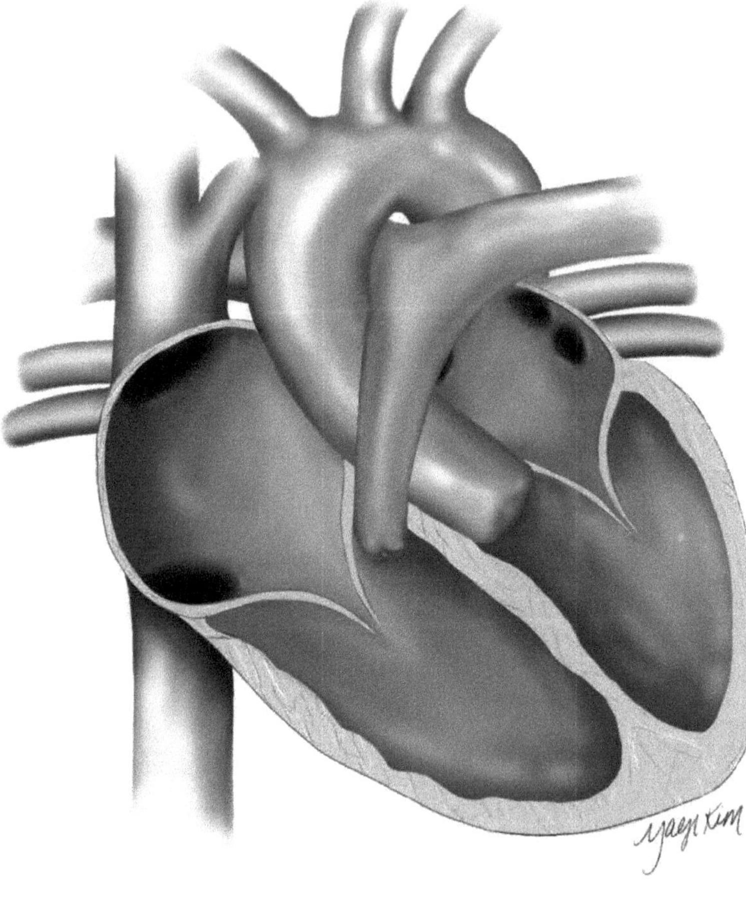

Limitation to pulmonary blood flow is characterized by a decreased amount of blood flow into the pulmonary circulation. This may be secondary to obstruction from stenosis or due to regurgitation.

With respect to the pulmonary circulation, pulmonary stenosis, subpulmonary stenosis, or right ventricular outflow tract obstruction can lead to impaired effective forward pulmonary blood flow.

Because the physiologic considerations and clinical management of stenosis and regurgitation differ, each will be addressed separately. Both can coexist. While left-to right or right-to-left shunts can occur in the setting of limitation to pulmonary blood flow, these will not be addressed here. The principles from the other sections can be layered on top of this framework. The arterial duct will be discussed here, as pulmonary blood flow may be ductal dependent. Atresia, such as pulmonary atresia with intact ventricular septum, will not be covered here as it aligns with functionally univentricular circulation which is discussed elsewhere.

Direction of blood flow: stenosis

In the setting of pulmonary blood flow limitation due to stenosis, the systemic circulation is generally preserved. Systemic venous return enters the right atrium, crosses the tricuspid valve into the right ventricle, and is pumped through the pulmonary valve into the pulmonary trunk and the branch pulmonary arteries.

With pulmonary valve stenosis, right ventricular outflow tract obstruction, or supravalvar pulmonary stenosis, forward flow into the pulmonary arteries is restricted. Blood that does not cross the obstruction remains in the right ventricle.

If an arterial duct is present, systemic blood flow can partially cross the duct into the pulmonary circulation, supplementing pulmonary blood flow. The direction and magnitude of ductal shunting depend on the relative resistances in the systemic and pulmonary circulations.

Distribution of blood flow into the pulmonary and systemic circulations: stenosis

In the absence of an arterial duct or shunt, systemic venous return and pulmonary blood flow are generally equal. This may not be the case in the setting of significant limitation to pulmonary blood flow. When the stenosis is mild, forward pulmonary blood flow is maintained, though at the expense of elevated right ventricular pressure. When the stenosis is severe, pulmonary blood flow may be diminished, and right atrial and right ventricular volume rises as blood is retained.

When an arterial duct is present, systemic output can be shared with the pulmonary circulation. If systemic resistance is greater than pulmonary resistance, systemic-to-pulmonary shunting across the duct can help augment pulmonary blood flow. If pulmonary vascular resistance is elevated, the contribution of the arterial duct to pulmonary blood flow may be limited.

Saturations: stenosis

The arterial oxygen saturation may decrease as pulmonary blood flow begins to get significantly limited, particularly if an atrial level shunt is present. In the setting of an arterial duct with systemic-to-pulmonary shunting, augmentation of blood flow can help improve the systemic arterial oxygen saturation.

The systemic venous oxygen saturation will depend on the adequacy of oxygen delivery. In the setting of hypoxemia, the oxygen extraction ratio will better reflect the adequacy of oxygen delivery rather than the arteriovenous oxygen saturation difference or the absolute venous saturation.

Pressures and volumes: stenosis

Stenosis increases right-sided pressures and volumes. The specific location dictates which chamber dilates over time.

Tricuspid valve stenosis leads to increased right atrial pressure and eventual right atrial dilation.

Right ventricular outflow tract obstruction leads to increased right ventricular systolic pressure and then eventually right ventricular dilation.

Pulmonary valve stenosis leads to elevated right ventricular systolic pressure and eventual right ventricular hypertrophy.

Over time, the right ventricle and right atrium may dilate depending on the severity of obstruction.

Clinical considerations in the context of the oximetric framework: stenosis

In the setting of limitation to pulmonary blood flow due to stenosis, widening arteriovenous oxygen saturation difference or increasing oxygen extraction ratio reflect decreasing adequacy of systemic oxygen delivery.

Increasing right ventricular contractility may help augment driving blood flow past right ventricular outflow tract obstruction but eventually may strain the right ventricle.

Preload augmentation may help support right ventricular filling and pulmonary blood flow, but excessive preload risks right-sided dilation and dysfunction.

Ductal patency can be essential to ensure pulmonary blood flow, particularly in severe stenosis. Prostaglandin or ductal stenting can help maintain ductal patency. In the setting of right ventricular tract obstruction, right ventricular outflow tract stenting is also a possibility.

Surgical or catheter-based interventions to relieve obstruction should be considered when systemic oxygen delivery cannot be maintained with medical therapy.

Direction of blood flow: regurgitation

With pulmonary regurgitation, the systemic circulation remains intact. Systemic venous return passes to the right atrium and then the right ventricle via the tricuspid valve. The right ventricle pumps the blood into the pulmonary trunk and the branch pulmonary arteries.

In the setting of tricuspid regurgitation, some of the blood pumped from the right ventricle returns to the right atrium by means of the tricuspid valve. In the setting of pulmonary regurgitation, some of the blood pumped by the right ventricle returns to the right ventricle. Thus, effective forward pulmonary blood flow is reduced, as a fraction of each stroke volume reenters the right atrium or right ventricle.

The left side of the circulation is usually normal with pulmonary venous blood returning to the left atrium and then going through the mitral valve to the left ventricle and then through the aortic valve to the aorta.

Distribution of blood flow into the pulmonary and systemic circulations: regurgitation

Systemic venous return generally equals pulmonary venous return although this does not hold true with worsening regurgitation. As effective pulmonary blood flow decreases with worsening regurgitation, the result is reduced pulmonary blood flow relative to systemic flow.

Saturations: regurgitation

Systemic arterial oxygen saturation may be reduced if there is enough limitation to pulmonary blood flow. Pulmonary venous saturation generally remains normal unless there is secondary parenchymal lung disease. Systemic venous oxygen saturation decreases with reduced adequacy of oxygen delivery.

Pressures and volumes: regurgitation

Regurgitation produces right ventricular volume overload and secondarily increases right-sided pressures. In the setting of tricuspid regurgitation there is an increase in right atrial pressure and volume while in the setting of pulmonary regurgitation there is an increase in right ventricular pressure and right ventricular volume.

Clinical considerations in the context of the oximetric framework: regurgitation

In the setting of pulmonary regurgitation, an increasing arteriovenous oxygen saturation difference or increasing oxygen extraction ratio indicates decreasing adequacy of systemic oxygen delivery due to reduced effective pulmonary blood flow.

Increasing contractility may augment systemic flow but also increases the regurgitant volume. Volume loading may worsen right ventricular dilation and function.

Afterload reduction has little role, as pulmonary resistance is not usually the limiting factor. Instead, therapies focus on maintaining right ventricular function are required.

Surgical interventions to limit regurgitation should be considered with systemic oxygen delivery cannot be maintained with medical therapy.

10
Limitation of systemic blood flow physiology

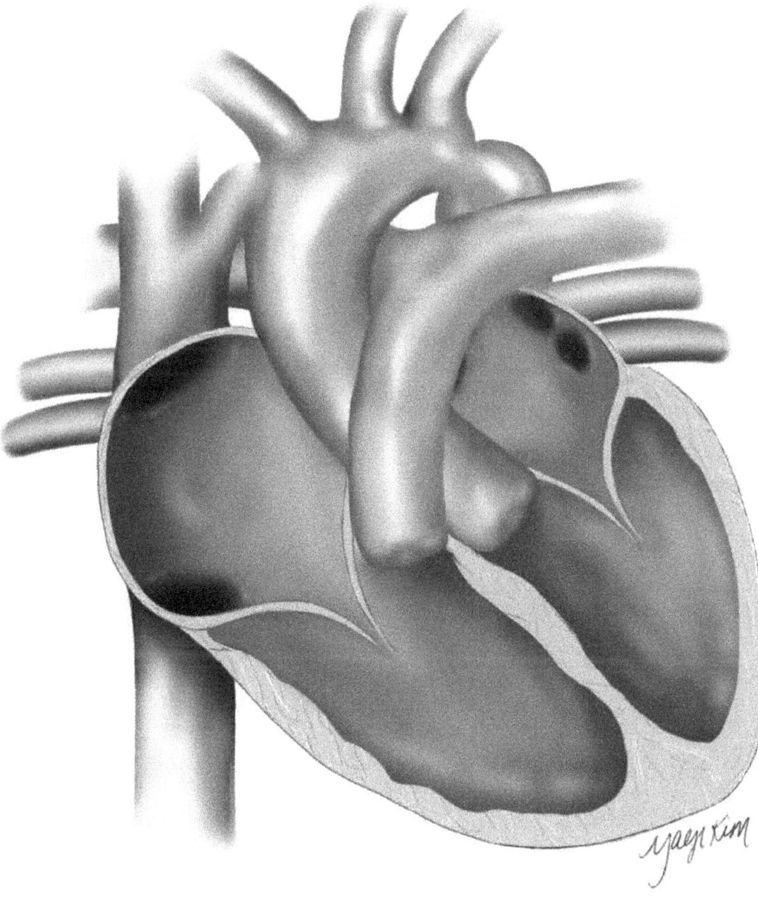

Limitation to systemic blood flow is characterized by reduced blood flow to the systemic circulation. This may be due to stenosis or regurgitation.

With respect to the systemic circulation, mitral stenosis, subaortic stenosis, left ventricular outflow tract obstruction from septal hypertrophy, aortic stenosis, supravalvar aortic stenosis, coarctation of the aorta, or interruption of the aortic arch can lead to limitation of systemic blood flow. In some of these settings, systemic blood flow may require a patent arterial duct. With respect to the systemic circulation, mitral regurgitation or aortic regurgitation may lead to limitation of systemic blood flow.

Since the physiologic considerations of, and clinical management of, stenosis and regurgitation vary, the chapter will address both individually. As with the circulatory physiologies themselves, both can occur simultaneously. While left to right shunts can occur in the setting of limitation of systemic blood flow, we will not address these here beyond the effects on the direction of blood flow. The principles from the left to right shunt physiology section can be layered on top of the considerations for limitation to systemic blood flow. This chapter, however, will address the arterial duct as systemic blood flow may be ductal dependent in this setting. Additionally, atresia of left sided structures, such as mitral or aortic atresia won't be covered in this chapter as those lend themselves to functionally univentricular physiology discussed elsewhere.

Direction of blood flow: stenosis

With limitation to systemic blood flow due to stenosis, the right sided circulation is generally not affected. There are generally usual systemic venous connections with the systemic venous return coming back to the right atrium and then entering the right ventricle via the tricuspid valve. Then this blood is pumped by the right ventricle to the pulmonary trunk via the pulmonary valve and then go to the branch pulmonary arteries.

This blood then returns to the left atrium via the pulmonary veins. If there is mitral stenosis, blood will still make its way to the left ventricle via the mitral valve although if there is an atrial level shunt there may be some right to left shunting across this. From the left ventricle the blood will be pumped into the aorta via the aortic valve. Subaortic stenosis, left ventricular outflow tract obstruction secondary to septal hypertrophy, aortic stenosis, or supravalvar aortic stenosis, may impact blood flow at this point although not necessarily its directionality. Once in the aorta, the blood will continue forward to the head and neck vessels or the body. If there is an arterial duct present then blood may shunt from the systemic circulation to the pulmonary circulation, form the pulmonary circulation to the systemic circulation, or bidirectionally depending on the relative resistances in the two circuits.

Distribution of blood flow into the pulmonary and systemic circulations: stenosis

In the setting of left sided stenosis without an arterial duct or intracardiac shunts then systemic venous and coronary sinus return equals pulmonary blood flow. Systemic blood flow may equal pulmonary blood flow although if the degree of stenosis becomes significant then some blood may remain in the left side of the heart and lead to dilation and systemic blood flow that is not equal to pulmonary blood flow. This can lead to dilation, pulmonary venous congestion, and ventricular dysfunction.

In the setting of left sided stenosis, obstruction to forward flow shifts the balance such that blood may preferentially enter the pulmonary circulation. The presence of an arterial duct can result in a situation where blood ejected from the right partially goes to the pulmonary circulation and partially to the systemic circulation, depending on the relative pulmonary and systemic pulmonary vascular resistances.

Saturations: stenosis

In a fully septated biventricular heart with left sided stenosis and no arterial duct, systemic arterial saturations will remain normal. When an arterial duct is present and there is shunting from the pulmonary to systemic circulations then there may be differential arterial saturations with preductal saturations being higher than postductal saturations. The postductal saturation will be the weighted average of the saturation of the pulmonary venous blood and the pulmonary arterial blood in this situation. In the setting of shunting from the systemic to pulmonary circulations via an arterial duct, the arterial saturations are generally normal.

Intracardiac saturations should be normal in the setting of a fully septated biventricular heart if systemic oxygen delivery is adequate. In the setting of inadequate systemic oxygen delivery then there will be systemic venous desaturation that will lead to lower than usual right sided saturations.

Pressures and volumes: stenosis

Stenosis leads to increased pressures. What structures experience this elevated pressure depends on the level of stenosis. When mitral stenosis is present, left atrial pressure rises. In the setting of aortic stenosis and coarctation, left ventricular pressure rises.

In the setting of mitral stenosis, the left atrial volume may increase with time, in the setting of aortic stenosis or coarctation, the left ventricle and left atrium may dilate with time.

Clinical considerations in the context of the oximetric framework: stenosis

In the setting of limitation to systemic blood flow due to stenosis, a widening arteriovenous oxygen saturation difference or increasing oxygen extraction ratio imply worsening adequacy of oxygen delivery. The primary reason for worsening adequacy of oxygen delivery is generally a decrease in cardiac output (systemic blood flow).

When the major components of oxygen delivery (oxygen extraction, oxygen content, heart rate, preload, afterload, contractility) are considered the special considerations in the setting come with respect to contractility and preload.

Modulating cardiac output in the setting of obstruction to systemic flow due to stenosis relies on contractility and preload. Contractility can help increase systemic flow. The degree of stenosis will not change but the amount of systemic flow may increase. Preload is also important for the heart in a situation like this where simply increasing how much is available for the heart to pump may promote contractility and also allow for more systemic blood flow. Fluid boluses must be given with close monitoring, however, especially in the setting of ventricular dysfunction. Afterload reduction in the setting of a fixed reduction is unlikely to help and will certainly increase the gradient across any obstruction although that doesn't necessarily mean that systemic flow has decreased.

Maintaining ductal patency may be important to help maximize systemic blood flow and can be done using prostaglandin or stenting the duct. Surgical systemic to pulmonary artery shunts can also be used of necessary.

Surgical intervention or catheter-based intervention should be considered when medical management is unable to maintain systemic oxygen delivery.

Direction of blood flow: regurgitation

In the setting of limitation to systemic blood flow due to regurgitation, the right sided circulation is generally not affected. There are generally usual systemic venous connections with the systemic venous return coming back to the right atrium and then entering the right ventricle via the tricuspid valve. Then this blood is pumped by the right ventricle to the pulmonary trunk via the pulmonary valve and then goes to the branch pulmonary arteries.

This blood then enters the left atrium via the pulmonary veins. Blood then enters the left ventricle via the mitral valve. From the left ventricle blood will enter the aorta via the aortic valve. If there is mitral regurgitation, some of the blood pumped by the left ventricle will also get ejected through the mitral valve and into the left atrium, eventually returning to the left ventricle. If there is aortic regurgitation, some of the blood pumped by the left ventricle through the aortic valve into the aorta will return to the left ventricle. Mitral regurgitation will occur during systole while aortic regurgitation will occur during diastole. In the setting of mitral or aortic regurgitation, part of the stroke volume is lost to regurgitant flow and effective forward systemic blood flow is reduced.

Distribution of blood flow into the pulmonary and systemic circulations: regurgitation

In the setting of mitral or aortic regurgitation, systemic venous return equal pulmonary venous return. However, because part of the left-sided stroke volume is contributed to a regurgitant circulation, effective systemic forward flow is reduced because some blood returns to the left ventricle. Thus, systemic blood flow is lower than pulmonary venous return.

Saturations: regurgitation

Systemic arterial oxygen saturation should be normal in the absence of parenchymal lung disease. In the setting of severe mitral regurgitation, significant pulmonary venous congestion may lead to pulmonary edema and lead to pulmonary venous desaturation and, subsequently, some arterial desaturation. Due to reduced systemic blood flow the venous oxygen saturation may be decreased, with a greater oxygen extraction ratio.

Pressures and volumes: regurgitation

Regurgitation increases volumes, and secondarily, pressures. Volume overload is generally isolated to the proximal chambers.

With mitral regurgitation, left atrial pressure rises during systole. Over time, left atrial volume increases and pulmonary venous pressures may rise. The left ventricle also dilated to accommodate the regurgitant volume in addition to the forward stroke volume.

With aortic regurgitation, left ventricular end-diastolic volume and pressure increase as blood reenters the ventricle from the aorta. This leads to left ventricular dilation and eccentric hypertrophy.

Clinical considerations in the context of the oximetric framework: regurgitation

In the setting of limitation to systemic blood flow due to regurgitation, a widening arteriovenous oxygen saturation difference or increasing oxygen extraction ratio imply worsening adequacy of oxygen delivery. This is generally the result of reduced effective systemic blood flow.

When considering the components of oxygen delivery, left ventricular end diastolic volume increases. This may improve left ventricular contractility but may lead to worsening pulmonary venous congestion or ventricular dilation.

Increasing contractility in the setting of regurgitation may increase systemic blood flow but it also increases the regurgitant volume (not necessarily fraction). Nonetheless, this may be helpful.

Afterload reduction is particularly important, as lowering systemic vascular resistance decreases the regurgitant fraction and, thus, promotes increased systemic blood flow.

Surgical intervention or catheter-based intervention should be considered when medical management is unable to maintain systemic oxygen delivery.

11
Transposition physiology

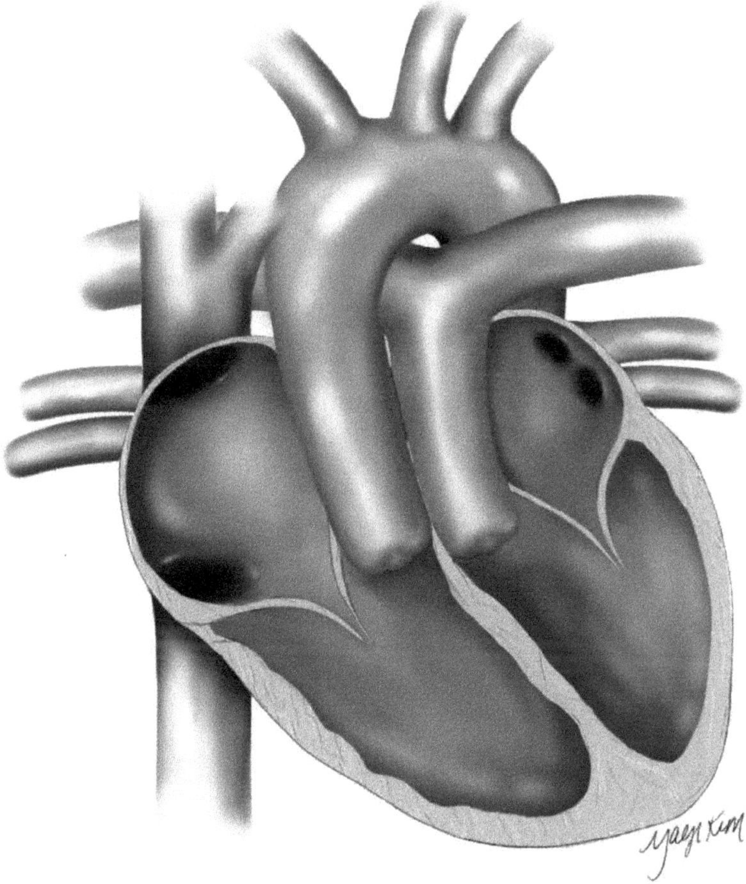

In the setting of transposition (discordant ventriculo-arterial connections) with an intact ventricular septum, the circulation is arranged in parallel rather than in series. The right atrium and the right ventricle receive systemic venous blood and direct it into the aorta, while the left atrium and ventricle receive pulmonary venous blood and direct it back into the pulmonary artery. Without sites of mixing, these two circuits remain entirely separate, and systemic oxygen delivery is progressively impaired. Survival therefore depends on the adequacy of mixing of the systemic venous and pulmonary venous blood pools, primarily at the atrial level, and secondarily at the arterial duct. This physiology produces a unique set of hemodynamic and oximetric considerations that differ from those in series circulation.

Outflow tract obstruction or a ventricular septal defect (left to right shunt) can coexist but as with previous circulatory physiologies this chapter will focus on transposition in its purest form. Concepts from other sections can be overlayed as needed.

Direction of blood flow

Systemic venous blood enters the right atrium, crosses the tricuspid valve into the right ventricle, and is pumped into the aorta. Pulmonary venous blood enters the left atrium, crosses the mitral valve into the left ventricle, and is pumped into the pulmonary artery. With an intact ventricular septum, there is no direct communication between the ventricles. Thus, only the atrial septum and the arterial duct provide sites for mixing to occur.

The atrial septum is the most efficient site of mixing, with both the size of the communication and the relative compliance of the atria determining the magnitude of mixing. When the atrial septum is restrictive, left atrial pressure rises, pulmonary venous return is obstructed, and pulmonary congestion results.

Distribution of blood flow into the pulmonary and systemic circulations

Because there are discordant ventriculo-arterial connections, distribution of blood into the systemic and pulmonary circulations depends on the sites of mixing present. In the setting of transposition with an intact ventricular septum, bidirectional shunting allows for adequate mixing of the systemic venous and pulmonary venous blood flows. In the setting of a restrictive atrial septum, most pulmonary venous return recirculates into the pulmonary circuit and systemic venous return recirculates into the systemic circuit. Thus, effective pulmonary blood flow (amount of deoxygenated blood going to the pulmonary circulation) is greatly reduced although absolute pulmonary blood flow may be normal or even high.

The arterial duct contributes to the distribution of blood flow most in the immediate newborn period, when pulmonary vascular resistance is elevated and pulmonary-to-systemic flow may help augment systemic flow and improve mixing at this level. As pulmonary vascular resistance decreases, arterial ductal flow tends to become more systemic-to-pulmonary, increasing pulmonary blood flow but adding little to systemic oxygen delivery.

The arterial duct, when present, increases blood flow into the pulmonary arteries if pulmonary vascular resistance is less than systemic vascular resistance. This leads to an increase in pulmonary venous return to the left atrium which increases left atrial volume and pressure, promoting more blood to go left to right at the atrial level. This mechanism allows for more oxygenated pulmonary venous blood to enter the systemic venous atrium, mix with the systemic venous blood pool, and reach the systemic circulation. In this way, ductal patency supports systemic oxygen delivery indirectly.

Saturations

Systemic arterial oxygen saturation in transposition depends on the degree of mixing between the systemic venous and pulmonary venous blood pools. With a restrictive atrial septum, systemic arterial oxygen saturations may be extremely low, as pulmonary venous blood cannot effectively enter the systemic circulation.

With an unrestrictive atrial septum, saturations are higher, though still below normal.

Mixing at the level of the arterial duct can also contribute although the arterial duct is a less efficient site of mixing.

The systemic venous oxygen saturation will depend on the arterial oxygen saturation as well as oxygen extraction. If the arteriovenous difference increases or the oxygen extraction ratio increases, this is indicative of worsening adequacy of systemic oxygen delivery.

"Shunting" in transposition

In transposition, the concept of a "net shunt" across any connection is not entirely accurate. Because the systemic and pulmonary circuits are arranged in parallel, any flow crossing at the atrial or ductal level drains one circuit and enters the other. Over the course of the cardiac cycle this results in mixing of the blood pools rather than a true net shunt in one direction. The magnitude of mixing is determined by the size and relative compliances of the chambers at the site of mixing. Thus, “shunting” or movement of blood in transposition must be equal in both directions and be fundamentally reciprocal, otherwise one circulation would be left emptied.

Pressures and volumes

In transposition, the right ventricle functions as the systemic ventricle and is pressure-loaded, generating systemic arterial pressures. The left ventricle functions as the pulmonary ventricle and is pressure-unloaded, generating only pulmonary arterial pressures. Without systemic afterload, the left ventricle may have a decrease in myocardial mass and thickness, limiting its ability to support the systemic circulation if repair is delayed.

At the atrial level, restriction of the oval fossa produces elevated left atrial pressure, pulmonary venous hypertension, and secondary pulmonary edema. The arterial duct, when patent, may reduce systemic diastolic pressure due to runoff into the pulmonary circulation once pulmonary vascular resistance decreases.

Special considerations

When the atrial septum is restrictive, left atrial pressure rises, pulmonary venous return is impeded, and pulmonary edema develops. Systemic oxygen delivery is critically reduced. This results in significant hypoxemia and acidemia.

If the arterial duct closes, this may reduce overall mixing of the systemic venous and pulmonary venous blood pools. With an unrestrictive atrial level shunt, systemic oxygen delivery may be adequate. With a restrictive atrial septum, ductal closure may lead to inadequate systemic oxygen delivery.

In the early days of life, elevated pulmonary vascular resistance permits some pulmonary to systemic shunt, allowing for augmentation of systemic blood flow and systemic oxygen delivery. As pulmonary resistance decreases, ductal shunting begins to reverse and there may not be as much contribution to the systemic circulation. Additionally, pulmonary blood flow increases.

Clinical considerations in the context of the oximetric framework

In the setting of transposition, systemic oxygen delivery is generally limited by the lack of adequate mixing of the systemic venous and pulmonary venous blood pools. Clinical management, thus, usually focuses on ensuring adequate mixing.

Maintaining ductal patency with prostaglandin infusion can help provide an additional site for mixing as well as allowing for increasing pulmonary blood flow, left atrial pressure, and consequently shunting of oxygenated blood from the left atrium to the systemic circulation. Balloon atrial septostomy may be considered when there is hypoxemia and a restrictive atrial septum. Modulating vascular resistances can transiently favor ductal shunting but this is less reliable once pulmonary vascular resistance declines.

Preload augmentation increases total cardiac output, increasing both the pulmonary and systemic blood flows.

Similarly, augmenting contractility increases total cardiac output, increasing both the pulmonary and systemic blood flows.

Transfusion can help by increasing oxygen content and thus increasing the systemic venous oxygen saturation. As there is mixing of the systemic venous and pulmonary venous blood pools, this results in a greater arterial oxygen saturation and greater systemic oxygen delivery as well.

Catheter-based or surgical interventions should be considered when medical management cannot help reliably maintain systemic oxygen delivery.

Problem	Oximetric Finding	Intervention	Goal
Inadequate mixing (restrictive atrial septum, duct closure)	Severe hypoxemia, ↑ extraction ratio	Prostaglandin infusion (maintain ductal patency)	Add site for mixing, support systemic DO_2
Restrictive atrial septum	Low SaO_2 despite ductus	Balloon atrial septostomy	Improve atrial mixing, reduce LA pressure
Declining systemic DO_2	Low SaO_2, ↓ SvO_2, ↑ extraction ratio	Transfusion	↑ O_2 content, raise SvO_2, ↑ mixed SaO_2
Limited total output	Low SvO_2, rising extraction	Preload augmentation, inotropes	↑ CO to both circuits
Progressive hypoxemia or inadequate DO_2 despite medical therapy	Oximetric indices not improving	Surgical intervention	Definitive separation of circuits

12
Functionally univentricular physiologies

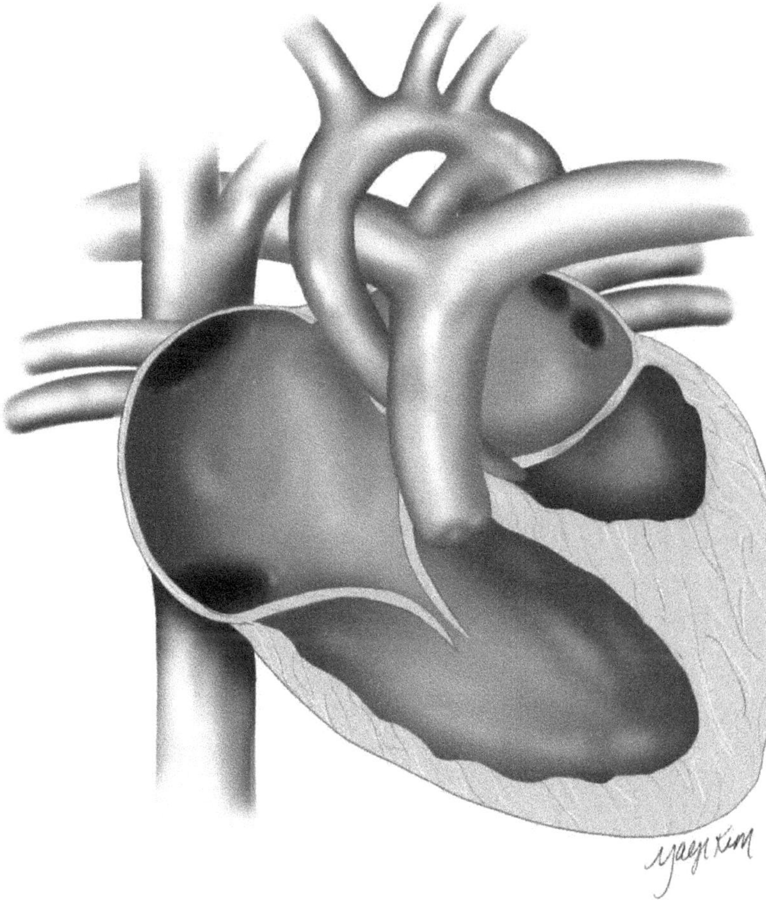

In functionally univentricular hearts, one ventricle is unable to support either the systemic or pulmonary circulation. In most of these hearts there are in fact two ventricles, anatomically, although one may be slit-like. There are some hearts with a solitary ventricle although these are rare. Hence, the term functionally univentricular is more appropriate.

In functionally univentricular hearts, all systemic venous and pulmonary venous return must be managed by a single ventricle. Surgical palliation consists of a series of potentially three surgical interventions (some may require additional surgical interventions) intended to separate the systemic and pulmonary blood flow. These surgeries are the Norwood operation, the Glenn operation, and the Fontan operation. Not all patients with functionally univentricular hearts will require a Norwood operation. Discussion of the specifics of each operation will not be covered here as this can be readily found elsewhere.

Through the course of this surgical palliation, there are different circulatory physiologies. There is no singular functionally univentricular physiology. There are three distinct circulatory physiologies: multidistributive physiology which exists prior to the Glenn operation, Glenn physiology which exists after the Glenn operation, and Fontan physiology which exists after the Fontan operation.

There are several nuances of each of these circulatory physiologies and this chapter is not meant to cover all the details of each of these circulations but to provide an overview and place it in the context of the oximetric framework. As before, there may be elements of other circulatory physiologies (limitation to pulmonary blood flow or limitation to systemic blood flow) but this chapter will cover the basics of the three physiologies and ignore coexistence of other circulatory physiologies.

Direction of blood flow: multidistributive physiology

In functionally univentricular multidistributive physiology, systemic venous blood enters the right atrium, passes through the atrioventricular valve into the systemic ventricle, and is pumped into both the aorta and the pulmonary arteries. Blood flow distribution depends on the relative resistances of the systemic and pulmonary circulations and on the patency of the arterial duct. Blood that enters the pulmonary circulation returns to the heart via the pulmonary veins. There is not, and cannot be, complete separation of the pulmonary and systemic circulations. Mixing of the systemic venous and pulmonary venous blood pools may occur at the atrial and/or ventricular level.

As blood with the same oxygen saturation (due to mixing of the systemic venous and pulmonary venous blood pools) is ejected from a functional single ventricle, the pumped blood can go to either the systemic or pulmonary circulation. Additionally, if there is atrioventricular valve regurgitation, some blood may get pumped to the atrium to return to the ventricle again. These are the different circulations that blood pumped by the ventricle can enter, hence the name of this circulatory physiology.

Distribution of blood flow: multidistributive physiology

The systemic ventricle generates the total cardiac output which is then divided into the pulmonary and systemic circulations. Thus, total cardiac output is the sum of pulmonary blood flow and systemic blood flow. If total cardiac output stays constant, any increase in pulmonary blood flow must be accompanied by an equal decrease in systemic blood flow, and vice versa. The relative distribution of blood flow to the pulmonary and systemic circulations is determined by the relative resistances of the two circulations. Increases in pulmonary blood flow must be met by decreases in systemic blood flow, if total cardiac output remains constant, and systemic blood flow and thus systemic oxygen delivery may become inadequate.

Using the Fick equation for pulmonary blood flow and systemic blood flow it becomes apparent that the ratio of pulmonary blood flow to systemic blood flow is equal to (arterial oxygen saturation – venous saturation) / (pulmonary venous saturation – pulmonary artery saturation). At the bedside it is important to note that in multidistributive physiology, arterial oxygen saturation and pulmonary artery saturation are equal. The venous saturation can be obtained by a venous blood gas or estimated using near infrared spectroscopy. This equation also highlights that the ratio of pulmonary to systemic blood flow cannot be assessed with an isolated systemic arterial oxygen saturation. At any given systemic arterial oxygen saturation, a wide range of pulmonary to systemic blood flow ratios are possible, depending on what the venous saturation is.

Saturations: multidistributive physiology

In functionally univentricular multidistributive physiology, the systemic arterial oxygen saturation represents a weighted average of the systemic venous and pulmonary venous oxygen saturations. The coefficients of this weighted average are determined by the relative amounts of pulmonary and systemic blood flow. Because pulmonary venous blood is nearly fully saturated, and is less variable from moment to moment, the arterial oxygen saturation is directly tied to the systemic venous oxygen saturation.

This relationship means that systemic arterial saturation is closely linked to the systemic venous saturation. A decrease in arterial oxygen saturation or in the systemic venous oxygen saturation must result in an obligatory decrease in the other in the next cardiac output, provided that systemic oxygen extraction remains the same or increases. This can lead to rapid development of significant inadequacy of systemic oxygen delivery when pulmonary blood flow decreases and/or systemic oxygen extraction rises. Thus, even small changes in the relative amounts of pulmonary and systemic blood flow or oxygen extraction can lead to profound desaturation.

Pressures and volumes: multidistributive physiology

In functionally univentricular multidistributive physiology, the systemic ventricle is markedly volume-loaded, receiving both systemic and pulmonary venous return. It pumps blood into both circulations, facing the combined impedance of the systemic and pulmonary vascular beds.

Clinical considerations in the context of the oximetric framework: multidistributive physiology

The adequacy of systemic oxygen delivery in functionally univentricular multidistributive physiology, like all physiologies discussed in this text, can be monitored using oxygen extraction. An increase in oxygen extraction implies a decrease in the adequacy of systemic oxygen delivery.

In this circulation, augmenting arterial oxygen content can help augment systemic oxygen delivery. This can be done by increase the fraction of inspired oxygen or by increasing the hemoglobin with a packed red blood cell transfusion. Anecdotally, there has been a fear of increasing the fraction of inspired oxygen in these patients as this could increase the pulmonary blood flow which could decrease systemic blood flow. Studies have demonstrated that while pulmonary blood flow does increase, so does systemic blood flow. Augmenting arterial oxygen content with fraction of inspired oxygen content can be done safely and monitoring oxygen extraction can indicate if it has become detrimental to systemic oxygen delivery.

Augmenting systemic venous oxygen content can also help augment systemic oxygen delivery. This can be done by increasing the hemoglobin with a packed red blood cell transfusion.

Preload augmentation can help increase total cardiac output, increasing both pulmonary and systemic blood flow. Preload augmentation can be accomplished with any intravenous fluid or blood product. Red blood cell transfusion can also help augment preload.

Afterload reduction can help increase systemic blood flow, and thus systemic oxygen delivery. Decreasing systemic vascular resistance relative to pulmonary vascular resistance can help promote more of the total cardiac output to go to the systemic circulation rather than the pulmonary circulation.

Contractility is important as it helps increase total cardiac output, increasing both pulmonary and systemic blood flow.

Heart rate is also an important consideration, particularly atrioventricular synchrony, as atrioventricular dyssynchrony can lead to a marked reduction in stroke volume in the setting of multidistributive physiology. Thus, maintaining atrioventricular synchrony can help optimize systemic oxygen delivery.

Direction of blood flow: Glenn physiology

After the superior cavopulmonary anastomosis, blood from the superior caval vein drains directly into the pulmonary arteries without a subpulmonary pump. The inferior caval vein drains into the atrium, mixes with pulmonary venous return, and then is ejected by the systemic ventricle into the systemic circulation.

Distribution of blood flow: Glenn physiology

In functionally univentricular Glenn physiology, total cardiac output now equals systemic blood flow. This differs from the situation in multidistributive physiology. Systemic blood flow consists of pulmonary venous return as well as inferior caval venous return. Pulmonary blood flow consists of superior caval venous return and any antegrade pulmonary blood flow that may have been left as well. Thus, pulmonary blood flow in Glenn physiology depends on the superior caval vein and pulmonary vascular resistance.

Saturations: Glenn physiology

In Glenn physiology, the system arterial oxygen saturation is a weighted average of the pulmonary venous oxygen saturation and the inferior caval venous oxygen saturation. As the superior caval venous return now goes directly to the lungs and gets oxygenated, there is less mixing than with multidistributive physiology. This does mean that there is less variability and greater stability in systemic arterial oxygen saturation.

Pressures and volumes: Glenn physiology

With Glenn physiology, the ventricle is partially volume unloaded relative to multidistributive physiology, since superior caval venous flow bypasses the systemic ventricle. As superior caval venous flow must make it through the pulmonary circulation without a pump, superior caval venous pressure must be elevated to help drive pulmonary flow, making the circulation highly sensitive to pulmonary vascular resistance.

Clinical considerations in the context of the oximetric framework: Glenn physiology

The adequacy of systemic oxygen delivery in functionally univentricular Glenn physiology, like all physiologies discussed in this text, can be monitored using oxygen extraction. An increase in oxygen extraction implies a decrease in the adequacy of systemic oxygen delivery.

In this circulation, augmenting systemic arterial oxygen content by increasing the fraction of inspired oxygen or via transfusion of packed red blood cells can help augment systemic oxygen delivery.

Augmenting systemic venous oxygen content via transfusion of packed red blood cells can help augment systemic oxygen delivery as there is still mixing of deoxygenated and oxygenated blood (inferior caval venous return and pulmonary venous return).

Preload is important in Glenn physiology as it impacts ventricular filling and stroke volume. In Glenn physiology, preload is also important as it establishes the driving pressure for pulmonary blood flow from the superior caval vein. Adequate intravascular volume is required to maintain superior caval vein pressure at a level sufficient to overcome pulmonary vascular resistance and sustain forward pulmonary blood flow. Excessive intravascular volume raises venous pressure without significantly improving flow so preload must be titrated to oximetric indices.

An additional clinical consideration unique to Glenn physiology is that the partial pressure of carbon dioxide impacts pulmonary venous oxygen saturation and thus systemic arterial oxygen saturation. Higher carbon dioxide levels promote cerebral vasodilation and increase cerebral blood flow. This results in greater superior caval venous return which is equal to pulmonary blood flow. Increased pulmonary blood flow helps augment the systemic arterial saturation. This is particularly important to keep in mind in patients with Glenn physiology who are intubated and mechanically ventilated.

Direction of blood flow: Fontan physiology

In functionally univentricular Fontan physiology, both superior and inferior caval venous blood flows return directly into the pulmonary arteries without a pump. The oxygenated blood returns to the atrium via the pulmonary veins and then returns to the systemic ventricle via the atrioventricular valve. The systemic ventricle receives only pulmonary venous return and pumps exclusively to the systemic circulation.

In some instances, a fenestration may be left in the Fontan which allows for some blood from the Fontan pathway (the inferior caval vein) to enter the atrium. Thus, there may be some mixing of the systemic venous and pulmonary venous blood pools, but this is minimal.

Distribution of blood flow: Fontan physiology

In Fontan physiology, pulmonary and systemic blood flows are generally equal in the absence of significant collaterals. Thus, total cardiac output equals systemic blood flow which equals pulmonary blood flow.

All systemic venous blood must pass through the lungs before entering the heart. Of course, the exception is if there is a fenestration then a small amount may go directly from the Fontan to the atrium. All pulmonary blood flow is passive, and preload dependent, driven by systemic venous pressure and limited by pulmonary vascular resistance. Any increase in pulmonary vascular resistance can reduce pulmonary blood flow, ventricular preload, and cardiac output.

Saturations: Fontan physiology

The systemic arterial oxygen saturation in the Fontan is usually near 100%, since all systemic venous return must pass through the lungs before entering the heart. The exception, once again, is a small amount of blood that can directly enter the atrium from the Fontan directly if there is a fenestration. While this can lead to some arterial desaturation it is minimal.

Pressures and volumes: Fontan physiology

The ventricle is volume-unloaded, receiving only pulmonary venous return, thus, systemic ventricular preload is reduced, limiting stroke volume relative to the Glenn physiology. Systemic venous pressure is chronically elevated to drive pulmonary blood flow, producing systemic venous hypertension.

Clinical considerations in the context of the oximetric framework: Fontan physiology

The adequacy of systemic oxygen delivery in functionally univentricular Fontan physiology, like all physiologies discussed in this text, can be monitored using the oxygen extraction ratio.

Since all pulmonary blood flow is passive and without a pump, maintaining adequate preload is of great importance as intravascular volume helps drive Fontan flow. Excessive preload, however, can lead to further increasing venous pressures and thus must be titrated carefully.

Fontan failure is characterized by high pressure in the Fontan circuit which limit pulmonary blood flow. These high venous pressures can impact pulmonary blood flow and the organs such as the liver and the kidneys.

Physiology	Flow Distribution	Arterial Saturation	Preload Consideration	Ventricular Load
Multidistributive	Single ventricle → Ao + PA (parallel)	Weighted mix of SvO_2 + PvO_2	Preload augments both Qp & Qs	Volume loaded
Glenn	SVC → PA, IVC+Pv → ventricle → Ao	Weighted mix (PvO_2 + IVC sat)	Preload drives SVC→PA flow	Partially unloaded
Fontan	SVC + IVC → PA (passive) → Pv → ventricle → Ao	Near 100% (except fenestration)	Preload essential but excessive preload → venous HTN	Volume unloaded, low preload

Physiology	Main Limitation	Key Monitoring	Key Interventions
Multidistributive	Reciprocal changes in Qp and Qs	Extraction ratio	FiO_2, Hb, preload, afterload modulation
Glenn	PVR-sensitive pulmonary flow	Extraction ratio, CO_2 levels	Maintain preload, modulate $PaCO_2$, transfusion
Fontan	Passive pulmonary flow, venous HTN	Extraction ratio	Maintain preload, avoid ↑ PVR

13
Ventricular dysfunction

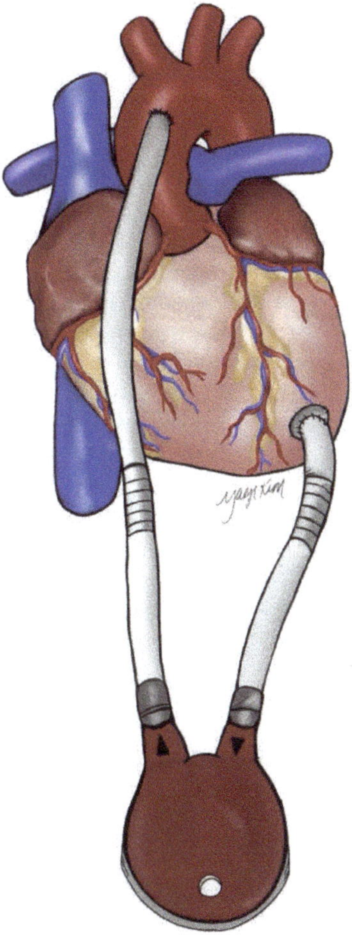

Ventricular dysfunction is a major determinant of systemic oxygen delivery. The ventricle provides the pressure and flow to help initiate systemic circulation, and when its function is impaired, systemic oxygen delivery may be compromised. Dysfunction may be present in the right and/or left ventricle and may consist of systolic and/or diastolic dysfunction. Each presents unique considerations.

Direction of blood flow

The direction of blood flow is normal in the setting of ventricular dysfunction. Systemic venous blood enters the right atrium and then goes to the right ventricle via the tricuspid valve. Ther right ventricle then pumps this blood into the pulmonary trunk via the pulmonary valve. Oxygenated blood returns from the lungs to the left atrium via the pulmonary veins and then goes to the left ventricle via the mitral valve. The left ventricle then pumps blood into the aorta via the aortic valve.

While the route of blood flow is maintained the issue in the setting of ventricular dysfunction is maintaining the amount of forward flow. In the setting of systolic dysfunction, forward systemic flow is directly reduced while in the setting of diastolic dysfunction, ventricular filling is restricted thus limiting stroke volume even in the setting of preserved contractility.

Distribution of blood flow

In the setting of left ventricular systolic and/or diastolic dysfunction, systemic blood flow is primarily affected. In the setting of right ventricular dysfunction, pulmonary blood flow is reduced which subsequently limits systemic blood flow. Thus, regardless of which ventricle is involved, systemic flow is impaired either directly or indirectly.

Pulmonary blood flow and systemic blood flow may not be equal, particularly as ventricular dysfunction progresses. In the setting of left ventricular dysfunction, pulmonary blood flow is often preserved initially because right ventricular function is intact, but systemic blood flow is reduced. Over time, rising left atrial pressure may reduce pulmonary venous return and limit pulmonary blood flow.

In the setting of right ventricular dysfunction, there is a direct decrease in pulmonary blood flow. This leads to reduced pulmonary venous return which means there is decreased left ventricular preload and thus decreased systemic blood flow.

Saturations

Systemic arterial oxygen saturation is usually normal. However, systemic venous oxygen saturation decreases due to inadequate systemic oxygen delivery.

Pressures and volumes

In left ventricular systolic dysfunction, left-sided filling pressures are elevated, leading to pulmonary venous hypertension and congestion. In left ventricular diastolic dysfunction, filling pressures are high despite normal or reduced ventricular volume.

In right ventricular dysfunction, right atrial and systemic venous pressures are elevated, producing venous congestion. Left-sided filling is reduced due to decreased left ventricular preload.

Clinical considerations in the context of the oximetric framework

The adequacy of systemic oxygen delivery in the setting of ventricular dysfunction, like all physiologies discussed in this text, can be monitored using oxygen extraction. The adequacy of systemic oxygen delivery can be variable across the spectrum of ventricular dysfunction. For instance, the same left ventricular ejection fraction or systemic blood flow may be adequate for a patient in a moment and then inadequate in a separate moment.

Intuitively, in the setting of systolic dysfunction, improving contractility can be particularly helpful. This can be done by use of inotropes.

Preload must be maintained to provide the right or left ventricle something to pump and to maintain stroke volume. However, excessive filling can worsen congestion.

Afterload reduction can strongly influence ventricular stroke volume in the setting of ventricular dysfunction and thus afterload reduction can be particularly helpful.

Heart rate may naturally increase to help the body maintain stroke volume but too high of a heart rate may reduce filling time, stroke volume, and subsequently systemic oxygen delivery. Decreasing heart rate and increasing diastolic filling time may help improve stroke volume and thus systemic oxygen delivery in the setting of ventricular dysfunction.

Mechanical circulatory support should be considered when medical management is unable to maintain systemic oxygen delivery.

14
Respiratory support and cardiopulmonary interactions

Gas exchange is fundamental for the maintenance of systemic oxygen delivery. Oxygen must be transferred from the atmosphere to the alveoli, diffuse across the alveolar-capillary membrane, and bind to the hemoglobin for transport in the systemic circulation. At the same time, carbon dioxide produced by metabolism must be eliminated. Within the oximetric framework, both oxygen uptake and carbon dioxide clearance are essential to maintaining the components of systemic oxygen delivery. Respiratory support, therefore, plays a central role in the care of critically ill children.

This chapter is not meant to cover all the details of respiratory support but is meant to highlight the basic physiologic and clinical principles and consider them in the context of the oximetric framework.

Oxygenation

The primary determinant of arterial oxygen content is hemoglobin saturation. Adequate oxygenation requires both delivery of oxygen to the alveoli and sufficient diffusion across the alveolar-capillary membrane. Respiratory support for oxygenation focuses on inspired oxygen concentration and mean airway pressure, which together govern alveolar oxygen tension and surface area available for gas exchange. Augmentation of the fraction of inspired oxygen increases alveolar oxygen tension and thereby enhances hemoglobin saturation.

This can be achieved by noninvasive means (such as conventional nasal cannula, high flow nasal cannula, continuous positive airway pressure, or bi-level positive airway pressure) or by invasive ventilation with an endotracheal tube. Airway oxygen concentration and pressure are less effectively augmented by noninvasive means.

From an oximetric perspective, ensuring that hemoglobin is adequately saturated is crucial, since systemic oxygen delivery is the product of arterial oxygen content and cardiac output. Thus, oxygenation strategies aim not only to maintain an acceptable systemic arterial oxygen saturation but to ensure that this is achieved in a manner that preserves systemic blood flow and avoids compromise of other components of systemic oxygen delivery.

Ventilation

Ventilation is essential for removing carbon dioxide, which is a major determinant of blood pH and thereby influences hemoglobin's affinity for oxygen. The key parameter is minute ventilation, determined by tidal volume and respiratory rate. Respiratory support for ventilation requires the delivery of positive pressure to augment the pressure gradient for gas flow.

With noninvasive respiratory support, positive pressure is delivered through an interface such as a mask or nasal prongs, and the achievable airway pressure is limited by comfort and leak. Invasive respiratory support, delivery via an endotracheal tube, allows greater control of airway pressure and tidal volumes. Respiratory support for ventilation must balance carbon dioxide clearance with the risk of excessive airway pressure or volumes, which may impede systemic blood flow and oxygen delivery.

Within the oximetric framework, maintaining appropriate ventilation ensures that systemic oxygen delivery is matched by systemic oxygen extraction and prevents the additional burden of acidosis on tissue oxygen utilization. Additionally, in the setting of significant respiratory distress, the respiratory muscles can use up to 35% of circulating oxygen. Thus, minimizing respiratory distress also helps reduce oxygen extraction, improving the adequacy of systemic oxygen delivery.

Cardiopulmonary interactions

Both negative and positive pressure ventilation influence systemic oxygen delivery by altering venous return, ventricular filling, and contractility. Negative pressure ventilation augments venous return and generally supports right ventricular and left ventricular preload.

Positive pressure ventilation has different effects on the right and left heart. The right ventricle is particularly sensitive to changes in intrathoracic pressure. Positive pressure ventilation increases pulmonary vascular resistance and reduces venous return, both of which may impair right ventricular output. This effect is further compounded in the setting of right ventricular dysfunction or elevated pulmonary vascular resistance, where even modest increases in airway pressure can significantly compromise pulmonary blood flow.

On the left side, positive pressure ventilation can decrease left ventricular afterload by reducing transmural pressure. This may help enhance systemic cardiac output in the setting of left ventricular dysfunction. While left ventricular afterload changes favorably with positive pressure ventilation, left ventricular preload changes unfavorably with positive pressure ventilation.

Within the oximetric framework, these cardiopulmonary interactions must always be considered, as even small shifts in intrathoracic pressure can alter the balance between systemic arterial oxygen saturation, cardiac output, and systemic oxygen delivery.

Clinical considerations in the context of the oximetric framework

Respiratory support cannot be viewed in isolation from the oximetric framework. Augmentation of the fraction of inspired oxygen, the balance of noninvasive and invasive strategies, the delivery of positive pressure for ventilation, and the effects of intrathoracic pressure on the heart all converge on the same goal: optimizing systemic oxygen delivery. Decisions about oxygenation, ventilation, and ventilatory mode must there be guided not only by gas exchange but also by their integrated effects on preload, afterload, contractility, and systemic blood flow.

15
Venous circulation

The venous circulation is often the least emphasized portion of the circulation, yet it is the largest volume compartment of the cardiovascular system. Venous return is what completes the loop- without it, systemic oxygen delivery cannot be maintained, no matter how well the heart pumps or how well gas exchange occurs.

What actually keeps blood flowing around the circulatory loop is not fully delineated, yet many assume that there are simple explanations for this. The heart clearly generates a pressure gradient, but whether that alone is sufficient to circulate blood is not entirely settled. Several different theories have been advanced, each providing insight but also facing important limitations.

This chapter will focus on the mystery of the venous circulation, highlighting current theories of how our circulatory system works but also highlighting that the precise mechanism of how the circulatory system works is still not entirely delineated.

Theories of venous return

Heart as the pump

The most intuitive view of the circulatory system is that the heart itself is the pump that propels blood through the circulation. Ventricular contraction clearly generates forward pressure and flow, and arterial pulsatility is an obvious demonstration of this. But this perspective fails to explain venous return for a key reason: the energy imparted by the heart is largely dissipated in the capillary network.

The arterioles and capillaries are the principal sites of resistance, where pulsatile energy is converted into steady flow and pressure drops dramatically. By the time blood traverses the capillary beds, very little of the kinetic energy from ventricular contraction remains. If venous return were simply the continuation of the heart's push, flow would be expected to stall once this energy was exhausted. Yet, venous blood reliably returns to the heart even in this low-pressure environment, and even during diastole when the heart is not actively contracting.

The limits of this theory are further underscored by environments such as microgravity or zero gravity, where blood still finds its way back to the heart without the aid of gravity. The limitations of this theory are also underscored by conditions of right atrial pressure elevation, where venous return is still partially preserved despite the diminished gradient. The heart is essential for circulation, but it is not sufficient to explain venous return.

Waterfall model

This model imagines the circulation like water spilling over a waterfall: once blood passes the arterioles, it flows downhill toward the right atrium under the influence of gravity. This waterfall analogy explains certain postural effects on venous return in humans. Yet, the model breaks down in species such as the giraffe. With necks several feet long, giraffes would face impossible hydrostatic challenges returning blood uphill from their heads if gravity alone dictated venous return. Similarly, in humans in space- where gravity is absent- venous return continues despite the absence of any "downhill" force. The waterfall model may apply in specific postures but cannot universally explain the circulation.

Siphon model

Others have suggested the circulation functions like a siphon: once blood is moving through a closed loop, it continues to flow as long as the loop is intact. This perspective highlights the circularity of blood flow and explains why flow persists without constant pumping effort. But siphons depend on rigid, uninterrupted columns of fluid, and veins do not behave this way. At low right atrial pressures, veins partially collapse, breaking the siphon analogy. Moreover, if circulation were purely a siphon, changes in gravity should not matter- yet we see fluid shifts in spaceflight and marked venous pooling in upright humans. The siphon captures the continuity of circulation but misses the collapsible nature of veins and the importance of venous pressure gradients.

Guyton's model: mean circulatory filling pressure and the two-compartment venous system

Arthur Guyton reframed the discussion of the venous system by focusing on mean circulatory filling pressure. He posited that venous return is governed by the gradient between mean circulatory filling pressure and right atrial pressure, where mean circulatory filling pressure represents the equilibrated pressure that would exist if the heart stopped and blood redistributed evenly. Mean circulatory filling pressure depends on both total blood volume and venous tone.

Guyton further described the venous system as two components: unstressed volume and stressed volume. Unstressed volume is the blood that fills the veins without exerting pressure while stressed volume is the blood that stretches the venous walls, generating pressure and driving venous return. By shifting blood from the unstressed to the stressed compartment- primarily through venoconstriction- mean circulatory filling pressure increases, and venous return rises. Venodilation does the reverse.

Guyton's framework also explains why circulation persists in settings that confound other theories. In the giraffe, high mean circulatory filling pressure combined with specialized venous valves allows venous return despite the vertical neck. In astronauts, where neither waterfall nor siphon models apply, venous return may be preserved because stressed volume still generates a pressure gradient toward the heart, even if the distribution shifts cephalad in microgravity. In this way, Guyton's model accounts for both terrestrial and extraterrestrial physiology, highlighting the venous system as an active regulator rather than passive plumbing.

Two compartment model

A complementary concept views the venous circulation as divided into two major compartments: the splanchnic venous circulation and the extra-splanchnic venous circulation. The splanchnic venous bed is large and highly compliant, functioning as a reservoir that holds a large proportion of total blood volume. The extra-splanchnic venous system consists of the non-splanchnic veins that return blood more directly to the heart.

Physiologically, the splanchnic venous system behaves as thought is partly in parallel and partly in series with the rest of the venous circulation. In parallel, because it is one of the multiple venous inflows to the right atrium; in series, because blood within this reservoir may need to be mobilized before it can contribute to central venous return.

This construct is clinically important as mobilization of splanchnic blood into the stressed compartment requires sympathetic activation or vasoactive medications. In shock states, much of the body's ability to recruit preload comes from shifting splanchnic volume. Conversely, in pathologic states such as sepsis, splanchnic venodilation traps blood in this compartment, lowering stressed volume and mean circulatory filling pressure despite normal or even elevated total blood volume.

Other contributors to venous return

Additional physiologic factors modify venous return. Skeletal muscle contraction can squeeze veins and propel blood forward, venous valves prevent retrograde flow, and intrathoracic pressure swings during respiration can augment or impede venous return depending on the phase of ventilation. These mechanisms modulate the pressure-flow relationships described by Guyton but are not primary determinants on their own.

Model	Core Idea	Key Limitation
Heart as pump	Ventricular contraction drives flow	Energy dissipated in capillaries, venous return persists even in diastole/microgravity
Waterfall	Gravity drives downhill flow	Fails in giraffe physiology and spaceflight
Siphon	Circulation as a closed-loop siphon	Veins collapse, gravity shifts not explained
Guyton's model	Venous return = MCFP – RA pressure	Hard to measure directly, but most comprehensive

Venous circulation in the oximetric framework

From the perspective of systemic oxygen delivery, the venous circulation serves as the reservoir that determines preload to the heart. It is not enough to think about the pump alone. Adequate stressed volume must be available and appropriately mobilized to maintain forward flow. When venous return is impaired- whether from low circulating volume, excessive venodilation, elevated right atrial pressure, or abnormal thoracic pressure swings- systemic oxygen delivery becomes less adequate, even if systemic arterial oxygen saturation and myocardial function preserved.

In the care of critically ill children this interplay is evident in several pathologic states. Venous congestion in heart failure illustrates how elevated right atrial pressure impairs venous return, reducing forward flow and systemic oxygen delivery even when systemic arterial oxygenation appears normal. Positive pressure ventilation can raise intrathoracic pressure and impede venous return, lowering preload and systemic oxygen delivery unless offset by adequate stressed volume. Sepsis with venodilation can reduce stressed volume, lowering mean circulatory filling pressure despite a normal or high total blood volume, leading to impaired return and low cardiac output. These clinical realities underscore that venous physiology is not abstract theory but central to daily management in critically ill children.

Venous saturations reflect this interplay. They provide insight into whether oxygen delivery and consumption are balanced, but also whether venous return itself is sufficient. Thus, the venous system is not simply passive plumbing but a dynamic determinant of systemic oxygen delivery in critically ill children.

Factor	Effect	Example
Volume status	↑ stressed volume → ↑ return	Fluid bolus
Venous tone	Constriction mobilizes stressed volume	Sepsis with venodilation
Right atrial pressure	↑ RAP → ↓ gradient → ↓ return	Heart failure with congestion
Intrathoracic pressure	↑ IT pressure → ↓ return	Positive pressure ventilation
Skeletal muscle/valves	Augment forward flow	Exercise, mobilization

16
The oximetric framework in practice

The oximetric framework provides a way to think about the care of critically ill children not through the lens of a pressure-based approach but through a complete and physiologically sound construct of systemic oxygen delivery. Each abnormal circulatory state described throughout this book ultimately challenges systemic oxygen delivery by impacting one or more of its component parts.

Systemic oxygen delivery depends on oxygen content and blood flow. Oxygen content is determined by hemoglobin concentration and systemic arterial oxygen saturation. Cardiac output depends on heart rate, preload, afterload, and contractility. Each circulatory physiology encountered in the pediatric cardiac intensive care unit can be dissected into which of these components is limited and what needs to be augmented.

Clinical thought process

When confronted with a child in shock or circulatory instability, the first step is to identify which component of systemic oxygen delivery is compromised: oxygen content, heart rate, preload, afterload, contractility.

The value of the oximetric framework lies in its universality. A child with aortic stenosis, a child after a Glenn operation, and a child in septic shock all appear clinically distinct, but each can be understood by identifying which component of systemic oxygen delivery is limited. This approach does not replace anatomic or diagnostic reasoning but complements it, integrating physiology, bedside observation, and therapeutic decision making.

By approaching care systematically, care becomes purposeful and targeted with interventions chosen to address specific physiologic limitation.

Conclusion

Clinical medicine is filled with complexity, but the underlying principles remain constant. The oximetric framework distills that complexity into a practical, reproducible method for guiding care. By focusing on systemic oxygen delivery and its components, clinicians can move past surface numbers and instead understand what is truly happening within the circulation. This clarity allows medical, surgical, or procedural interventions to be deployed with intention, precision, and the greatest possible benefit to the child being cared for.

References

These are simply representative references. This is not an exhaustive list of all pertinent publications. This should help guide you in the right direction to "trust but verify".

Reference regarding the oximetric framework
[1–5]

References regarding the value of monitoring oximetric indices
[6–18]

References regarding the relationship between NIRS and venous saturation
[11, 19–21]

Reference regarding the clinical utility of NIRS
[20–52]

References regarding serum lactate
[13, 53–57]

References regarding vasoactive support and vasodilators in non-cardiac arrest pediatric patients
[58–128]

References regarding the effects of cardiopulmonary bypass
[129–131]

References regarding blood transfusions
[132–136]

1. Loomba RS (2023) The Oximetric Approach to Clinical Care. Pediatr Cardiol 44:960–961. https://doi.org/10.1007/s00246-023-03127-8
2. Loomba RS, Flores S (2022) Oximetry titrated care: This is the way. Paediatr Anaesth 32:485. https://doi.org/10.1111/pan.14350

3. Karlsson J, Lönnqvist P-A (2022) Blood pressure and flow in pediatric anesthesia: An educational review. Paediatr Anaesth 32:10–16. https://doi.org/10.1111/pan.14328

4. Ferreira FM, Araujo DD, Dantas GM, et al (2025) Goal-directed therapy with continuous SvcO2 monitoring in pediatric cardiac surgery: the PediaSat single-center randomized trial. Brazilian Journal of Anesthesiology (English Edition) 75:844614. https://doi.org/10.1016/j.bjane.2025.844614

5. Loomba RS (2025) Venous saturation guided postoperative care for pediatric cardiac surgical patients: the body wants oxygen! Brazilian Journal of Anesthesiology (English Edition) 75:844641. https://doi.org/10.1016/j.bjane.2025.844641

6. Hoffman GM, Mussatto KA, Brosig CL, et al (2005) Systemic venous oxygen saturation after the Norwood procedure and childhood neurodevelopmental outcome. J Thorac Cardiovasc Surg 130:1094–1100. https://doi.org/10.1016/j.jtcvs.2005.06.029

7. Eliasdottir TS, Bragason D, Hardarson SH, et al (2015) Venous oxygen saturation is reduced and variable in central retinal vein occlusion. Graefes Arch Clin Exp Ophthalmol 253:1653–1661. https://doi.org/10.1007/s00417-014-2849-2

8. Takano H, Matsuda H, Kadoba K, et al (1994) Monitoring of hepatic venous oxygen saturation for predicting acute liver dysfunction after Fontan operations. J Thorac Cardiovasc Surg 108:700–708

9. Crowley R, Sanchez E, Ho JK, et al (2011) Prolonged central venous desaturation measured by continuous oximetry is associated with adverse outcomes in pediatric cardiac surgery. Anesthesiology 115:1033–1043. https://doi.org/10.1097/ALN.0b013e318233056e

10. Hirai N, Saito J, Nakai K, et al (2023) Association between regional oxygen saturation and central venous saturation in pediatric patients undergoing cardiac surgery: A prospective observational study. Paediatr Anaesth 33:913–922. https://doi.org/10.1111/pan.14741
11. Loomba RS, Rausa J, Sheikholeslami D, et al (2022) Correlation of Near-Infrared Spectroscopy Oximetry and Corresponding Venous Oxygen Saturations in Children with Congenital Heart Disease. Pediatr Cardiol 43:197–206. https://doi.org/10.1007/s00246-021-02718-7
12. McQuillen PS, Nishimoto MS, Bottrell CL, et al (2007) Regional and central venous oxygen saturation monitoring following pediatric cardiac surgery: concordance and association with clinical variables. Pediatr Crit Care Med 8:154–160. https://doi.org/10.1097/01.PCC.0000257101.37171.BE
13. Ranucci M, Isgrò G, Carlucci C, et al (2010) Central venous oxygen saturation and blood lactate levels during cardiopulmonary bypass are associated with outcome after pediatric cardiac surgery. Crit Care 14:R149. https://doi.org/10.1186/cc9217
14. Rossi AF, Sommer RJ, Lotvin A, et al (1994) Usefulness of intermittent monitoring of mixed venous oxygen saturation after stage I palliation for hypoplastic left heart syndrome. Am J Cardiol 73:1118–1123. https://doi.org/10.1016/0002-9149(94)90293-3
15. Samadi M, Malaki M, Ghaffari S, Golshan Khalili R (2012) Correlation Between Pediatric Open Heart Surgery Outcomes and Arterial-mixed Venous Oxygen Saturation Differences. J Cardiovasc Thorac Res 4:41–44. https://doi.org/10.5681/jcvtr.2012.010
16. Teele SA, Gazit AZ, Futterman C, et al (2025) Investigation of a Novel Noninvasive Risk Analytics Algorithm With Laboratory Central Venous Oxygen Saturation Measurements in Critically Ill Pediatric

Patients. Crit Care Explor 7:e1204. https://doi.org/10.1097/CCE.0000000000001204
17. Scott JP, Hoffman GM (2014) Near-infrared spectroscopy: exposing the dark (venous) side of the circulation. Paediatr Anaesth 24:74–88. https://doi.org/10.1111/pan.12301
18. Goonasekera CDA, Carcillo JA, Deep A (2018) Oxygen Delivery and Oxygen Consumption in Pediatric Fluid Refractory Septic Shock During the First 42 h of Therapy and Their Relationship to 28-Day Outcome. Front Pediatr 6:314. https://doi.org/10.3389/fped.2018.00314
19. Iliopoulos I, Flores S, Loomba R (2025) Near infrared spectroscopy in the pediatric cardiac intensive care unit: accurately interpreting the data. Curr Opin Cardiol 40:282–289. https://doi.org/10.1097/HCO.0000000000001204
20. Gil-Anton J, Redondo S, Garcia Urabayen D, et al (2015) Combined Cerebral and Renal Near-Infrared Spectroscopy After Congenital Heart Surgery. Pediatr Cardiol 36:1173–1178. https://doi.org/10.1007/s00246-015-1139-z
21. Hansen JH, Schlangen J, Armbrust S, et al (2013) Monitoring of regional tissue oxygenation with near-infrared spectroscopy during the early postoperative course after superior cavopulmonary anastomosis. Eur J Cardiothorac Surg 43:e37-43. https://doi.org/10.1093/ejcts/ezs581
22. Law MA, Benscoter AL, Borasino S, et al (2022) Inferior and Superior Vena Cava Saturation Monitoring After Neonatal Cardiac Surgery. Pediatr Crit Care Med 23:e347–e355. https://doi.org/10.1097/PCC.0000000000002963
23. Holleran EM, Brown MD, Sassano C, et al (2024) Monitoring abdominal near-infrared spectroscopy during feeds in neonates with CHD recovering from surgery: a

feasibility study. Cardiol Young 34:2355–2361. https://doi.org/10.1017/S1047951124036114

24. Tume LN, Arnold P (2015) Near-infrared spectroscopy after high-risk congenital heart surgery in the paediatric intensive care unit. Cardiol Young 25:459–467. https://doi.org/10.1017/S1047951114000055

25. Xie W, Liu Y, Zeng Y, et al (2024) Utilizing mesenteric near-infrared reflectance spectroscopy to predict gastrointestinal complication risks and optimize feeding strategies in infants undergoing cardiac surgery. Pediatr Investig 8:287–294. https://doi.org/10.1002/ped4.12437

26. Zulueta JL, Vida VL, Perisinotto E, et al (2013) Role of intraoperative regional oxygen saturation using near infrared spectroscopy in the prediction of low output syndrome after pediatric heart surgery. J Card Surg 28:446–452. https://doi.org/10.1111/jocs.12122

27. Zheng SC, He S (2025) The near-infrared spectroscopy to evaluate neonatal improvement after transfusion: a systematic review and meta-analysis. BMC Pediatr 25:385. https://doi.org/10.1186/s12887-025-05731-4

28. Troncoso G, Agudelo-Pérez S, Botero-Rosas D, et al (2025) Association between cerebral oxygen saturation and neurological injury in asphyxiated neonates in a middle-income country: a retrospective cohort study. BMJ Paediatr Open 9:e003081. https://doi.org/10.1136/bmjpo-2024-003081

29. Chen J, Fan X, He S, et al (2025) Regional tissue oxygen saturation during minimal enteral feeding is associated with the subsequent feeding intolerance in very preterm infants. Sci Rep 15:8558. https://doi.org/10.1038/s41598-025-92185-4

30. Aksoy M, Memur Ş, Yasa B, Çetinkaya M (2025) A Novel and Promising Method for Prediction of Early

Surfactant Requirement in Preterm Infants With Respiratory Distress Syndrome: Pulmonary Near-Infrared Spectroscopy. Pediatr Pulmonol 60:e71023. https://doi.org/10.1002/ppul.71023
31. Verhoeven R, Kupers T, Brunsch CL, et al (2024) Using Vital Signs for the Early Prediction of Necrotizing Enterocolitis in Preterm Neonates with Machine Learning. Children (Basel) 11:1452. https://doi.org/10.3390/children11121452
32. Kakajiwala A, Kamath N, Nesargi S, et al (2025) The use of near-infrared spectroscopy to measure kidney oxygenation in the neonatal intensive care unit. Pediatr Nephrol. https://doi.org/10.1007/s00467-025-06792-4
33. Condit PE, Gorski DP, Lasarev MR, et al (2024) Decreased Intraoperative Renal Tissue Oxygenation after Cardiopulmonary Bypass Predicts Cardiac Surgery-Associated Acute Kidney Injury in Neonates. Children (Basel) 11:315. https://doi.org/10.3390/children11030315
34. Inoue T, Kohira S, Ebine T, et al (2022) Monitoring of intraoperative femoral oxygenation predicts acute kidney injury after pediatric cardiac surgery. Int J Artif Organs 45:981–987. https://doi.org/10.1177/03913988221119527
35. Flechet M, Güiza F, Scharlaeken I, et al (2019) Near-Infrared-Based Cerebral Oximetry for Prediction of Severe Acute Kidney Injury in Critically Ill Children After Cardiac Surgery. Crit Care Explor 1:e0063. https://doi.org/10.1097/CCE.0000000000000063
36. Sinner B, Banas M, Brunete-Lorenzo C, et al (2020) Acute Kidney Injury and Renal Regional Oxygen Saturation During Pediatric Liver Transplantation. Ann Transplant 25:e919717. https://doi.org/10.12659/AOT.919717
37. Adams PS, Vargas D, Baust T, et al (2019) Associations of Perioperative Renal Oximetry Via Near-

Infrared Spectroscopy, Urinary Biomarkers, and Postoperative Acute Kidney Injury in Infants After Congenital Heart Surgery: Should Creatinine Continue to Be the Gold Standard? Pediatr Crit Care Med 20:27–37. https://doi.org/10.1097/PCC.0000000000001767

38. Joffe R, Al Aklabi M, Bhattacharya S, et al (2018) Cardiac Surgery-Associated Kidney Injury in Children and Renal Oximetry. Pediatr Crit Care Med 19:839–845. https://doi.org/10.1097/PCC.0000000000001656

39. Gist KM, Kaufman J, da Cruz EM, et al (2016) A Decline in Intraoperative Renal Near-Infrared Spectroscopy Is Associated With Adverse Outcomes in Children Following Cardiac Surgery. Pediatr Crit Care Med 17:342–349. https://doi.org/10.1097/PCC.0000000000000674

40. Ruf B, Bonelli V, Balling G, et al (2015) Intraoperative renal near-infrared spectroscopy indicates developing acute kidney injury in infants undergoing cardiac surgery with cardiopulmonary bypass: a case-control study. Crit Care 19:27. https://doi.org/10.1186/s13054-015-0760-9

41. Hazle MA, Gajarski RJ, Aiyagari R, et al (2013) Urinary biomarkers and renal near-infrared spectroscopy predict intensive care unit outcomes after cardiac surgery in infants younger than 6 months of age. J Thorac Cardiovasc Surg 146:861-867.e1. https://doi.org/10.1016/j.jtcvs.2012.12.012

42. Owens GE, King K, Gurney JG, Charpie JR (2011) Low renal oximetry correlates with acute kidney injury after infant cardiac surgery. Pediatr Cardiol 32:183–188. https://doi.org/10.1007/s00246-010-9839-x

43. Sood ED, Benzaquen JS, Davies RR, et al (2013) Predictive value of perioperative near-infrared spectroscopy for neurodevelopmental outcomes after cardiac surgery in infancy. J Thorac Cardiovasc Surg

145:438-445.e1; discussion 444-445. https://doi.org/10.1016/j.jtcvs.2012.10.033
44. Ghidini F, Benetti E, Zucchetta P, et al (2021) Transcutaneous near-infrared spectroscopy (NIRS) for monitoring kidney and liver allograft perfusion. Int J Clin Pract 75:e14034. https://doi.org/10.1111/ijcp.14034
45. Shiba J, Satoh M, Taira K, et al (2018) Near-infrared spectroscopy might be a useful tool for predicting the risk of vascular complications after pediatric liver transplants: Two case reports. Pediatr Transplant 22:. https://doi.org/10.1111/petr.13089
46. Colak M, Ceylan G, Topal S, et al (2023) Evaluation of renal near-infrared spectroscopy for predicting extubation outcomes in the pediatric intensive care setting. Front Pediatr 11:1326550. https://doi.org/10.3389/fped.2023.1326550
47. Savorgnan F, Loomba RS, Flores S, et al (2023) Descriptors of Failed Extubation in Norwood Patients Using Physiologic Data Streaming. Pediatr Cardiol 44:396–403. https://doi.org/10.1007/s00246-022-03084-8
48. Gradidge EA, Grimaldi LM, Cashen K, et al (2019) Near-infrared spectroscopy for prediction of extubation success after neonatal cardiac surgery. Cardiol Young 29:787–792. https://doi.org/10.1017/S1047951119000829
49. Foster CB, Spaeder MC, McCarter RJ, et al (2013) The use of near-infrared spectroscopy during an extubation readiness trial as a predictor of extubation outcome. Pediatr Crit Care Med 14:587–592. https://doi.org/10.1097/PCC.0b013e31828a8964
50. Loomba RS, Sheth SP, Wong J, et al (2025) Changes in adequacy of splanchnic oxygen delivery and splanchnic artery Doppler after bolus feedings in infants: A systematic review and meta-analysis. Pediatr Neonatol 66:272–277. https://doi.org/10.1016/j.pedneo.2024.04.014

51. Elhoff JJ, Acosta S, Flores S, et al (2024) Parental holding of infants improves haemodynamics in the cardiac ICU. Cardiol Young 34:1004–1009. https://doi.org/10.1017/S1047951123003931

52. Loomba RS, Dyamenahalli U, Savorgnan F, et al (2023) The effect of clinical and haemodynamic variables on post-operative length of stay immediately upon admission after biventricular repair with Yasui operation following an earlier Norwood operation. Cardiol Young 33:2066–2071. https://doi.org/10.1017/S1047951122003948

53. Asfari A, Wolovits J, Gazit AZ, et al (2023) A Near Real-Time Risk Analytics Algorithm Predicts Elevated Lactate Levels in Pediatric Cardiac Critical Care Patients. Crit Care Explor 5:e1013. https://doi.org/10.1097/CCE.0000000000001013

54. Klee P, Rimensberger PC, Karam O (2020) Association Between Lactates, Blood Glucose, and Systemic Oxygen Delivery in Children After Cardiopulmonary Bypass. Front Pediatr 8:332. https://doi.org/10.3389/fped.2020.00332

55. Loomba RS, Villarreal EG, Klein A, et al (2025) Poor correlation of venous lactate with systemic oxygen saturation in the paediatric cardiac ICU: a pilot study. Cardiol Young 35:157–161. https://doi.org/10.1017/S1047951124026805

56. Rocha VHS, Manso PH, Carmona F (2021) Central Venous Oxygen Saturation/Lactate Ratio and Prediction of Major Adverse Events After Pediatric Heart Surgery. Braz J Cardiovasc Surg 36:736–742. https://doi.org/10.21470/1678-9741-2020-0521

57. Loomba RS, Mansukhani S, Wong J (2024) Factors that mediate change in creatinine and acute kidney injury after the Norwood operation: insights from high-fidelity haemodynamic monitoring data. Cardiol

Young 34:1779–1786.
https://doi.org/10.1017/S1047951124000842
58. Loomba RS, Savorgnan F, Acosta S, et al (2024) Clinical Interventions and Hemodynamic Monitoring in the Setting of Left Ventricular Systolic Heart Failure in Children: Insights From a Physiologic Simulator. Am J Ther 31:e531–e540.
https://doi.org/10.1097/MJT.0000000000001711
59. Farias JS, Villarreal EG, Flores S, et al (2021) Effects of Vasopressin Infusion After Pediatric Cardiac Surgery: A Meta-analysis. Pediatr Cardiol 42:225–233.
https://doi.org/10.1007/s00246-020-02496-8
60. Loomba RS, Patel RD, Villarreal EG, et al (2024) Epinephrine Versus Dopamine in Children, What Is the Current Evidence and What Do We Need? A Systematic Review and Meta-analysis. J Pediatr Pharmacol Ther 29:578–586. https://doi.org/10.5863/1551-6776-29.6.578
61. Bronicki RA, Acosta S, Savorgnan F, et al (2022) The acute influence of vasopressin on hemodynamic status and tissue oxygenation following the Norwood procedure. JTCVS Open 9:217–224.
https://doi.org/10.1016/j.xjon.2022.01.008
62. Hendon E, Kane J, Golem GM, et al (2022) Acute effects of vasoactive medications in patients with parallel circulation awaiting hybrid or Norwood procedure. Ann Pediatr Cardiol 15:34–40.
https://doi.org/10.4103/apc.apc_39_21
63. Villarreal EG, Flores S, Kriz C, et al (2020) Sodium nitroprusside versus nicardipine for hypertension management after surgery: A systematic review and meta-analysis. J Card Surg 35:1021–1028.
https://doi.org/10.1111/jocs.14513
64. Loomba RS, Flores S (2019) Use of vasoactive agents in postoperative pediatric cardiac patients:

Insights from a national database. Congenit Heart Dis 14:1176–1184. https://doi.org/10.1111/chd.12837
65. Sun Y-T, Wang L-H, Yao Y-T, Evidence in Cardiovascular Anesthesia (EICA) Group (2025) Vasoactive-inotropic agents in pediatric patients undergoing cardiac surgery: A single-center retrospective study. Medicine (Baltimore) 104:e42333. https://doi.org/10.1097/MD.0000000000042333
66. Burkhardt BE, Hummel J, Rücker G, Stiller B (2024) Inotropes for the prevention of low cardiac output syndrome and mortality for paediatric patients undergoing surgery for congenital heart disease: a network meta-analysis. Cochrane Database Syst Rev 11:CD013707. https://doi.org/10.1002/14651858.CD013707.pub2
67. Loomba RS, Ikeda N, Farias JS, et al (2025) Comorbidities, pharmacologic interventions, and mechanical interventions associated with mortality in isolated diastolic left heart failure: lessons from a national database. Cardiol Young 35:102–108. https://doi.org/10.1017/S1047951124026787
68. Loomba RS, Savorgnan F, Acosta S, et al (2024) Clinical Interventions and Hemodynamic Monitoring in the Setting of Left Ventricular Systolic Heart Failure in Children: Insights From a Physiologic Simulator. Am J Ther 31:e531–e540. https://doi.org/10.1097/MJT.0000000000001711
69. Loomba RS, Villarreal EG, Farias JS, et al (2024) Factors associated with renal oxygen extraction in mechanically ventilated children after the Norwood operation: insights from high fidelity haemodynamic data. Cardiol Young 1–6. https://doi.org/10.1017/S1047951124025174
70. Joshi RK, Joshi R, Aggarwal N, et al (2024) Comparison of Levosimendan Versus Milrinone After the Arterial Switch Operation for Infants ≤3 kg. World J Pediatr

Congenit Heart Surg 15:588–596. https://doi.org/10.1177/21501351241239306
71. Matsushita FY, Krebs VLJ, de Campos CV, et al (2024) Reassessing the role of milrinone in the treatment of heart failure and pulmonary hypertension in neonates and children: a systematic review and meta-analysis. Eur J Pediatr 183:543–555. https://doi.org/10.1007/s00431-023-05342-0
72. Saengsin K, Sperotto F, Lu M, et al (2023) Administration of Milrinone Following Tetralogy of Fallot Repair Increases Postoperative Volume Administration Without Improving Cardiac Output. Anesth Analg 137:1056–1065. https://doi.org/10.1213/ANE.0000000000006662
73. Shao W, Diao S, Zhou L, Cai L (2023) Milrinone for the treatment of heart failure caused by severe Pneumonia in children with congenital heart disease: a meta-analysis. BMC Pediatr 23:537. https://doi.org/10.1186/s12887-023-04360-z
74. Prajapati M, Patel J, Patel H, et al (2022) Assessment of the effect of two regimens of milrinone infusion in paediatric patients with pulmonary artery hypertension undergoing corrective cardiac procedure: A prospective observational study. Ann Pediatr Cardiol 15:358–363. https://doi.org/10.4103/apc.apc_230_21
75. Soliman R, Ragheb A (2018) Assessment of the effect of two regimens of milrinone infusion in pediatric patients undergoing fontan procedure: A randomized study. Ann Card Anaesth 21:134–140. https://doi.org/10.4103/aca.ACA_160_17
76. Brown S, Nolan O, Poole E, et al (2023) Long-term milrinone therapy in children with dilated cardiomyopathy. Acta Paediatr 112:1298–1303. https://doi.org/10.1111/apa.16738

77. Beshish AG, Aljiffry A, Aronoff E, et al (2023) Milrinone for treatment of elevated lactate in the pre-operative newborn with hypoplastic left heart syndrome. Cardiol Young 33:1691–1699. https://doi.org/10.1017/S1047951122003171
78. Lapere M, Rega F, Rex S (2022) Levosimendan in paediatric cardiac anaesthesiology: A systematic review and meta-analysis. Eur J Anaesthesiol 39:646–655. https://doi.org/10.1097/EJA.0000000000001711
79. Jothinath K, Balakrishnan S, Raju V, et al (2021) Clinical efficacy of levosimendan vs milrinone in preventing low cardiac output syndrome following pediatric cardiac surgery. Ann Card Anaesth 24:217–223. https://doi.org/10.4103/aca.ACA_160_19
80. Kanazawa T, Shimizu K, Iwasaki T, et al (2021) Perioperative Milrinone Infusion Improves One-Year Survival After the Norwood-Sano Procedure. J Cardiothorac Vasc Anesth 35:2073–2078. https://doi.org/10.1053/j.jvca.2021.02.017
81. Hoffman GM, Niebler RA, Scott JP, et al (2021) Interventions Associated With Treatment of Low Cardiac Output After Stage 1 Norwood Palliation. Ann Thorac Surg 111:1620–1627. https://doi.org/10.1016/j.athoracsur.2020.05.068
82. Thorlacius EM, Wåhlander H, Ojala T, et al (2020) Levosimendan Versus Milrinone for Inotropic Support in Pediatric Cardiac Surgery: Results From a Randomized Trial. J Cardiothorac Vasc Anesth 34:2072–2080. https://doi.org/10.1053/j.jvca.2020.02.027
83. Loomba RS, Dorsey V, Villarreal EG, Flores S (2020) The effect of milrinone on hemodynamic and gas exchange parameters in children. Cardiol Young 30:55–61. https://doi.org/10.1017/S1047951119002865
84. Cavigelli-Brunner A, Hug MI, Dave H, et al (2018) Prevention of Low Cardiac Output Syndrome After

Pediatric Cardiac Surgery: A Double-Blind Randomized Clinical Pilot Study Comparing Dobutamine and Milrinone. Pediatr Crit Care Med 19:619–625. https://doi.org/10.1097/PCC.0000000000001533

85. Mills KI, Kaza AK, Walsh BK, et al (2016) Phosphodiesterase Inhibitor-Based Vasodilation Improves Oxygen Delivery and Clinical Outcomes Following Stage 1 Palliation. J Am Heart Assoc 5:e003554. https://doi.org/10.1161/JAHA.116.003554

86. Bianchi MO, Cheung P-Y, Phillipos E, et al (2015) The Effect of Milrinone on Splanchnic and Cerebral Perfusion in Infants With Congenital Heart Disease Prior to Surgery: An Observational Study. Shock 44:115–120. https://doi.org/10.1097/SHK.0000000000000388

87. Lee J, Kim GB, Kwon HW, et al (2014) Safety and efficacy of the off-label use of milrinone in pediatric patients with heart diseases. Korean Circ J 44:320–327. https://doi.org/10.4070/kcj.2014.44.5.320

88. Farah P, Ahmad-Ali A, Hanane G, Abbas E (2013) Additive effect of phosphodiesterase inhibitors in control of pulmonary hypertension after congenital cardiac surgery in children. Iran J Pediatr 23:19–26

89. Duggal B, Pratap U, Slavik Z, et al (2005) Milrinone and low cardiac output following cardiac surgery in infants: is there a direct myocardial effect? Pediatr Cardiol 26:642–645. https://doi.org/10.1007/s00246-005-0881-z

90. Hoffman TM, Wernovsky G, Atz AM, et al (2003) Efficacy and safety of milrinone in preventing low cardiac output syndrome in infants and children after corrective surgery for congenital heart disease. Circulation 107:996–1002. https://doi.org/10.1161/01.cir.0000051365.81920.28

91. Hoffman TM, Wernovsky G, Atz AM, et al (2002) Prophylactic intravenous use of milrinone after cardiac

operation in pediatrics (PRIMACORP) study. Prophylactic Intravenous Use of Milrinone After Cardiac Operation in Pediatrics. Am Heart J 143:15–21. https://doi.org/10.1067/mhj.2002.120305

92. Ramamoorthy C, Anderson GD, Williams GD, Lynn AM (1998) Pharmacokinetics and side effects of milrinone in infants and children after open heart surgery. Anesth Analg 86:283–289. https://doi.org/10.1097/00000539-199802000-00011

93. Eisenberg MA, Georgette N, Baker AH, et al (2025) Epinephrine vs Norepinephrine as Initial Treatment in Children With Septic Shock. JAMA Netw Open 8:e254720. https://doi.org/10.1001/jamanetworkopen.2025.4720

94. Garegrat R, Patnaik S, Suryawanshi S, et al (2024) A pilot randomized controlled trial comparing noradrenaline and adrenaline as a first-line vasopressor for fluid-refractory septic shock in neonates. Front Pediatr 12:1443990. https://doi.org/10.3389/fped.2024.1443990

95. Hasson DC, Gist KM, Seo J, et al (2024) The Association Between Vasopressin and Adverse Kidney Outcomes in Children and Young Adults Requiring Vasopressors on Continuous Renal Replacement Therapy. Crit Care Explor 6:e1156. https://doi.org/10.1097/CCE.0000000000001156

96. Wen L, Xu L (2020) The efficacy of dopamine versus epinephrine for pediatric or neonatal septic shock: a meta-analysis of randomized controlled studies. Ital J Pediatr 46:6. https://doi.org/10.1186/s13052-019-0768-x

97. Ross CE, Asaro LA, Wypij D, et al (2018) Physiologic response to pre-arrest bolus dilute epinephrine in the pediatric intensive care unit. Resuscitation 126:137–142. https://doi.org/10.1016/j.resuscitation.2018.03.011

98. Reiter PD, Roth J, Wathen B, et al (2018) Low-Dose Epinephrine Boluses for Acute Hypotension in the PICU. Pediatr Crit Care Med 19:281–286. https://doi.org/10.1097/PCC.0000000000001448
99. Achuff B-J, Achuff JC, Park HH, et al (2018) Epinephrine syringe exchange events in a paediatric cardiovascular ICU: analysing the storm. Cardiol Young 28:409–415. https://doi.org/10.1017/S1047951117002232
100. Ventura AMC, Shieh HH, Bousso A, et al (2015) Double-Blind Prospective Randomized Controlled Trial of Dopamine Versus Epinephrine as First-Line Vasoactive Drugs in Pediatric Septic Shock. Crit Care Med 43:2292–2302. https://doi.org/10.1097/CCM.0000000000001260
101. McFerson MC, McCanta AC, Pan Z, et al (2014) Tachyarrhythmias after the Norwood procedure: relationship and effect of vasoactive agents. Pediatr Cardiol 35:668–675. https://doi.org/10.1007/s00246-013-0836-8
102. Heckmann M, Trotter A, Pohlandt F, Lindner W (2002) Epinephrine treatment of hypotension in very low birthweight infants. Acta Paediatr 91:566–570. https://doi.org/10.1080/080352502753711704
103. Laitinen P, Happonen JM, Sairanen H, et al (1999) Amrinone versus dopamine and nitroglycerin in neonates after arterial switch operation for transposition of the great arteries. J Cardiothorac Vasc Anesth 13:186–190. https://doi.org/10.1016/s1053-0770(99)90085-x
104. Habib DM, Padbury JF, Anas NG, et al (1992) Dobutamine pharmacokinetics and pharmacodynamics in pediatric intensive care patients. Crit Care Med 20:601–608. https://doi.org/10.1097/00003246-199205000-00010
105. Vedrenne-Cloquet M, Chareyre J, Léger P-L, et al (2022) Low Dosing Norepinephrine Effects on Cerebral Oxygenation and Perfusion During Pediatric Shock. Front

Pediatr 10:898444.
https://doi.org/10.3389/fped.2022.898444

106. Gupta S, Agrawal G, Thakur S, et al (2022) The effect of norepinephrine on clinical and hemodynamic parameters in neonates with shock: a retrospective cohort study. Eur J Pediatr 181:2379–2387.
https://doi.org/10.1007/s00431-022-04437-4

107. Ranjit S, Natraj R, Kandath SK, et al (2016) Early norepinephrine decreases fluid and ventilatory requirements in pediatric vasodilatory septic shock. Indian J Crit Care Med 20:561–569.
https://doi.org/10.4103/0972-5229.192036

108. Piva J, Alquati T, Garcia PC, et al (2014) Norepinephrine infusion increases urine output in children under sedative and analgesic infusion. Rev Assoc Med Bras (1992) 60:208–215.
https://doi.org/10.1590/1806-9282.60.03.008

109. Eldadah MK, Schwartz PH, Harrison R, Newth CJ (1991) Pharmacokinetics of dopamine in infants and children. Crit Care Med 19:1008–1011.
https://doi.org/10.1097/00003246-199108000-00006

110. Zaritsky A, Lotze A, Stull R, Goldstein DS (1988) Steady-state dopamine clearance in critically ill infants and children. Crit Care Med 16:217–220.
https://doi.org/10.1097/00003246-198803000-00002

111. Pazandak C, McPherson C, Abubakar M, et al (2020) Blood Pressure Profiles in Infants With Hypoxic Ischemic Encephalopathy (HIE), Response to Dopamine, and Association With Brain Injury. Front Pediatr 8:512.
https://doi.org/10.3389/fped.2020.00512

112. Hotta M, Hirata K, Nozaki M, et al (2020) Association between amount of dopamine and infections in extremely preterm infants. Eur J Pediatr 179:1797–1803.
https://doi.org/10.1007/s00431-020-03676-7

113. Kirupakaran K, de Sousa P, Le Roux C, et al (2020) Evaluation of the causal effects between dopamine infusion changeover and fluctuations in mean arterial pressure in neonates. Arch Dis Child 105:390–394. https://doi.org/10.1136/archdischild-2019-317123

114. Baske K, Saini SS, Dutta S, Sundaram V (2018) Epinephrine versus dopamine in neonatal septic shock: a double-blind randomized controlled trial. Eur J Pediatr 177:1335–1342. https://doi.org/10.1007/s00431-018-3195-x

115. Seri I, Abbasi S, Wood DC, Gerdes JS (1998) Regional hemodynamic effects of dopamine in the sick preterm neonate. J Pediatr 133:728–734. https://doi.org/10.1016/s0022-3476(98)70141-6

116. Hentschel R, Hensel D, Brune T, et al (1995) Impact on blood pressure and intestinal perfusion of dobutamine or dopamine in hypotensive preterm infants. Biol Neonate 68:318–324. https://doi.org/10.1159/000244252

117. Seri I, Tulassay T, Kiszel J, et al (1984) Cardiovascular response to dopamine in hypotensive preterm neonates with severe hyaline membrane disease. Eur J Pediatr 142:3–9. https://doi.org/10.1007/BF00442581

118. Kwapisz MM, Neuhäuser C, Scholz S, et al (2009) Hemodynamic effects of dobutamine and dopexamine after cardiopulmonary bypass in pediatric cardiac surgery. Paediatr Anaesth 19:862–871. https://doi.org/10.1111/j.1460-9592.2009.03101.x

119. Li J, Zhang G, Holtby H, et al (2006) Adverse effects of dopamine on systemic hemodynamic status and oxygen transport in neonates after the Norwood procedure. J Am Coll Cardiol 48:1859–1864. https://doi.org/10.1016/j.jacc.2006.07.038

120. Lang P, Williams RG, Norwood WI, Castaneda AR (1980) The hemodynamic effects of dopamine in infants after corrective cardiac surgery. J Pediatr 96:630–634. https://doi.org/10.1016/s0022-3476(80)80727-x
121. Iliopoulos I, Flores S, Coghill M, et al (2025) Endocrine Effects of Arginine-Vasopressin After Pediatric Cardiac Surgery. Pediatr Cardiol. https://doi.org/10.1007/s00246-025-04049-3
122. Kumar A, Ghotra GS, Raj S, et al (2023) Low-Dose vasopressin and renal perfusion in pediatric cardiac surgery. Ann Card Anaesth 26:309–317. https://doi.org/10.4103/aca.aca_182_22
123. Mastropietro CW, Miletic K, Chen H, Rossi NF (2014) Effect of corticosteroids on arginine vasopressin after pediatric cardiac surgery. J Crit Care 29:982–986. https://doi.org/10.1016/j.jcrc.2014.07.007
124. Das S, Das D, Dutta N, et al (2025) Vasopressin as a postoperative management strategy in Fontan procedure: a comparative study. Indian J Thorac Cardiovasc Surg 41:395–403. https://doi.org/10.1007/s12055-024-01873-9
125. Loomba RS, Culichia C, Schulz K, et al (2021) Acute Effects of Vasopressin Arginine Infusion in Children with Congenital Heart Disease: Higher Blood Pressure Does Not Equal Improved Systemic Oxygen Delivery. Pediatr Cardiol 42:1792–1798. https://doi.org/10.1007/s00246-021-02667-1
126. Farias JS, Villarreal EG, Flores S, et al (2021) Effects of Vasopressin Infusion After Pediatric Cardiac Surgery: A Meta-analysis. Pediatr Cardiol 42:225–233. https://doi.org/10.1007/s00246-020-02496-8
127. Lu Z, Wang X, Yang J, et al (2018) Vasopressin in Vasodilatory Shock for Both Left and Right Heart Anomalous Pediatric Patients After Cardiac Surgery.

Shock 50:173–177.
https://doi.org/10.1097/SHK.0000000000001051
128. Burton GL, Kaufman J, Goot BH, da Cruz EM (2011) The use of Arginine Vasopressin in neonates following the Norwood procedure. Cardiol Young 21:536–544. https://doi.org/10.1017/S1047951111000370
129. Kozik DJ, Tweddell JS (2006) Characterizing the inflammatory response to cardiopulmonary bypass in children. Ann Thorac Surg 81:S2347-2354.
https://doi.org/10.1016/j.athoracsur.2006.02.073
130. Ashraf S (1997) Effects of cardiopulmonary bypass on neonatal and paediatric inflammatory profiles. European Journal of Cardio-Thoracic Surgery 12:862–868.
https://doi.org/10.1016/S1010-7940(97)00261-3
131. Chew MS, Brandslund I, Brix-Christensen V, et al (2001) Tissue Injury and the Inflammatory Response to Pediatric Cardiac Surgery with Cardiopulmonary Bypass: A Descriptive Study. Anesthesiology 94:745–753.
https://doi.org/10.1097/00000542-200105000-00010
132. Zuo Y, Zhang H, Lv L, et al (2025) Blood Transfusions are Associated With Prolonged Mechanical Ventilation Following Cardiac Surgery in Neonates. Rev Cardiovasc Med 26:36566.
https://doi.org/10.31083/RCM36566
133. Schiller O, Pula G, Shostak E, et al (2024) Patient-tailored platelet transfusion practices for children supported by extracorporeal membrane oxygenation. Vox Sang 119:326–334. https://doi.org/10.1111/vox.13583
134. Mikulski MF, Linero A, Stromberg D, et al (2024) Analysis of haemodynamics surrounding blood transfusions after the arterial switch operation: a pilot study utilising real-time telemetry high-frequency data capture. Cardiol Young 34:1109–1116.
https://doi.org/10.1017/S104795112400009X

135. Kuo JA, Maher KO, Kirshbom PM, Mahle WT (2011) Red blood cell transfusion for infants with single-ventricle physiology. Pediatr Cardiol 32:461–468. https://doi.org/10.1007/s00246-011-9901-3
136. Patel RD, Weld J, Flores S, et al (2022) The Acute Effect of Packed Red Blood Cell Transfusion in Mechanically Ventilated Children after the Norwood Operation. Pediatr Cardiol 43:401–406. https://doi.org/10.1007/s00246-021-02735-6

www.ingramcontent.com/pod-product-compliance
Lightning Source LLC
LaVergne TN
LVHW050936210926
848482LV00013B/628

* 9 7 9 8 3 4 9 6 9 3 9 6 0 *